Managing Challenges for the Flint Water Crisis

MANAGING CHALLENGES

FOR

THE FLINT WATER CRISIS

EDITED BY

TONYA E. THORNTON,
ANDREW D. WILLIAMS,
KATHERINE M. SIMON

AND

JENNIFER F. SKLAREW

Westphalia Press
An Imprint of the Policy Studies Organization
Washington, DC
2021

MANAGING CHALLENGES FOR THE FLINT WATER CRISIS

All Rights Reserved © 2021 by Policy Studies Organization

Westphalia Press
An imprint of Policy Studies Organization
1527 New Hampshire Ave., NW
Washington, D.C. 20036
info@ipsonet.org

ISBN: 978-1-63723-701-4

Cover and interior design by Jeffrey Barnes
jbarnesbook.design

Daniel Gutierrez-Sandoval, Executive Director
PSO and Westphalia Press

Updated material and comments on this edition
can be found at the Westphalia Press website:
www.westphaliapress.org

We dedicate this volume to the importance of effective governance in risk reduction and emergency management for all those working on emergency management in the twenty-first century.

It is our hope and belief that scholarship can connect with communities of practice—that is, public administrators, emergency managers, and first responders—as well as citizens, to serves as force multipliers in emergency planning and disaster response. It is they who should be recognized as a relevant means to ideological bridge building that strengthens social cohesion and political confidence, so that a more effective and integrated approach to community resiliency can be developed.

And to the memory of Paul L. Posner, whose life's work as a self-professed "pracademic" contributed immeasurably to good governance.

CONTENTS

PREFACE

In April 25, 2014, city officials began examining ways to save the city money. This was in direct response to the State of Michigan having taken over the City of Flint's finances, given that an audit in 2011 resulted in a projected $25 million deficit. Their solution was to switch Flint, Michigan's drinking water supply from the Detroit city system to the Flint River.

Two years prior, on March 22, 2012, Genesee County had announced a new pipeline was being designed to deliver water from Lake Huron to Flint. The plan was to reduce costs by switching the city's water supplier from the Detroit Water and Sewerage Department to the Karegnondi Water Authority. Then, just a year later, on April 16, 2013, per the city council's recommendation, Andy Dillon, the state's treasurer, authorized the City of Flint to make the switch to Flint River water. That switch occurred a little over a week later, on April 25, 2014.

At the time, Mayor Dayne Walling said, "Here's to Flint," as he lifted a glass filled with tap water in a celebratory manner. He walked along with other city and state officials who were toasting the switch of the city's drinking water source from Detroit's water system to the Flint River. Yet Flint was an aging industrial city with failing critical infrastructure, including the water piping system. It did not take long for residents to note differences in the water quality, and reports of dark-colored and foul-tasting and smelling water.

This new water from the Flint River was highly corrosive. And, even today, concerns still exist around the water crisis that continues to plague Flint, Michigan. Residents remain left with feelings of uncertainty given their intensive experience with the crisis: namely E. Coli outbreaks and lead spikes in blood levels.

The complexity of this crisis is squarely rooted in environmental science, public health, emergency management, and fiscal austerity. Bureaucratic complications remain to this day.

Concerns over transparency and accountability still rattle the local government, even with heavy-handed assistance from the state and federal governments. As of last fall, in August 2019, the State of Michigan warned City of Flint officials that Flint was in violation of the Safe Drinking Water Act because it failed to treat the water properly; lead leached out from aging pipes into thousands of homes.

Water is an essential source of life. It is, in fact, a critical resource.

Critical infrastructure supports lifeline systems that are considered essential to the successful functioning of governance and society in the United States (U.S.). They are the common thread that touches every public service delivery challenge of the future, across all levels of government. The efficient delivery of government services relies on a power grid functioning at full capacity, an operational and expansive communication network, a streamlined and efficient transportation system, and water infrastructure delivering clean and affordable water free of pollution ... all of which ensure public safety and national security.

The capacity and equity of these systems are pressing problems for all sectors—public, private, and nonprofit. The destruction of, or even inconsistency in, these systems would have a debilitating impact upon the economic vitality of the nation. Additionally, if such networks are disrupted, there will be a lasting impact upon the social cohesion and political trust of the community. Prioritizing the physical and operational condition of these systems will promote a sense of resiliency and ensure the necessities for human development that extend beyond traditional physiological and safety needs.

Systems are vulnerable, not just people. Critical infrastructure is considered essential to the successful functioning of governance and society in the U.S. Many discussions often center on the efficient delivery of government services relying upon a power grid functioning at full capacity—grids that power many of the other systems, such as operational and expansive communication, transportation, and water networks. If one system goes down, it will have a cascading effect upon the others.

Still, there is no coherent definition of system resiliency among the public and private sectors. Additionally, many systems have been underfunded and pose risks to lifelines due to damage from the elements, high-impact events, aging, and being outpaced by growing demand and technological advancements they can no longer support. More users and rising demand push or exceed infrastructure design capacity.

Safe drinking water is a prerequisite for protecting public health and all human activity, and properly treated wastewater is vital for preventing disease and protecting the environment. Ensuring the continuity of clean drinking water and wastewater treatment and service is essential to modern life and the nation's economy.

The current human capital environment is marked by efforts to build the next generation of public servants. Across the nation, the intergovernmental intersections between state and local governments are both contracting and growing. At the same time, in the midst of government draw-downs and budget cut-backs, cities and their leaders are innovating, advancing their communities into the next era of governance, and providing more effective and equitable public services.

This edited volume discusses a number of multidisciplinary issues that have not been previously examined concerning the Flint Water Crisis, including the social sciences, administrative and policy sciences, and community resiliency.

ACKNOWLEDGEMENTS

There are many individuals who have contributed to the success of this edited volume. Bonnie Stabile, Ph.D., an Associate Professor with George Mason University's Schar School of Policy and Government, should be thanked for the initial commissioning of this study. It has been a long time in the making.

We would also be remiss not to thank the many graduate research assistants at the Schar School who took time in assisting with the review process as well as editing and formatting. Those individuals include: Charles "Tyler" Goodwin, Ashley Raphael, Blanca Dionne-Rand, Grace Royer, Nicole Decker, Caroline Egli, Michael Sweigart, and Fleciah Mburu.

The study has also benefited greatly from the contributions of many individuals, who have compiled the respective chapters. They all have been generous in providing the scientific perspective required in examining such a complex issue that is multidisciplinary in nature. Many of these individuals are active members of the American Society of Public Administration and its Section on Emergency and Crisis Management.

MANAGING THE CRISIS

Anna Clark

Let me tell you a bit about a city that I love.

Flint is full of bright, smart, passionate people. One reason that this Michigan city has had an outsized impact on history is because its residents have a long tradition of community organizing. You see this turn up in all sorts of ways. There is General Motors, of course. Flint is the birthplace of the company that spent 77 years as the worldwide leader in auto sales. GM made extraordinary leaps forward in how both corporations and automobiles are designed, to say nothing of its wartime contributions to the "Arsenal of Democracy." But equally important is the 1936 - 1937 Sit Down Strike, through which workers won the right to collectively bargain. This made Flint the de facto birthplace of the United Auto Workers, which cued a nationwide push for labor rights that transformed the twentieth century.

Community education was also born in Flint during the Great Depression. This was an influential movement that imagined "lighted schoolhouses" serving as neighborhood hubs that not only provided K-12 education, but also adult classes, recreation, dental care, and other social services well into the evening hours.

As Flint's population boomed in the twentieth century, fueled by the Great Migration, tensions escalated over the city's staunch segregation. Racial apartheid was the policy and in practice at every level of civic life. It took years of organizing—not to mention a sleep-in at City Hall and a 5,000-person rally—but in 1968, by scarcely three dozen votes, Flint became the first city in America to pass a fair housing ordinance by popular vote.

Today's Flint is also a county seat, home to four college campuses, two major medical centers, and the second-largest art museum in the state. A farmer's market thrives in an old printing plant. Over on West Court Street, at a place called Totem, you'll find good coffee, books, music, and food, including the J-Worth sandwich, named after a resident who is a favorite customer. Hang out long at Totem's counter, and you'll have more interesting conversations than you'll know what to do with.

I want to share all this with you, and much more, because so often, Flint is spoken about *solely* in terms of loss. Over the decades, it has lost population, industry, jobs, schools, public services, and local democracy. The toll is incalculably large. At the same time, the litany of loss can obscure what is alive in Flint. This is a *place* we're talking about. Not a theory, not "ruin porn," but a city with a unique history, full of real people living real lives.

So let us begin there. Flint, this Great Lakes city with a history of punching above its weight, learned that its drinking water was toxic. Residents had to discover it themselves, in fact. As the water worsened with each passing day and concerns about quality fell on deaf ears, residents did the work themselves of sharing knowledge, canvassing doors, hosting bottled water deliveries, mapping symptoms, and coordinating with outside experts to gather more and better data than what any other agency was providing. It showed that yes, this was a citywide drinking water crisis, and yes, it had been seriously hurting people all along, despite official assurances otherwise. Lead poisoning, especially for children, has permanent and incurable consequences, and the two-year outbreak of Legionnaire's disease—not disclosed by public officials until after the national spotlight turned on Flint in 2016—killed people.

Here in a state that is surrounded by more than 20 percent of all the freshwater on the planet's surface, caution tape went up over drinking fountains. Hydrants pumped out brown liquid in an attempt to clear the corroded pipes. Parents were warned about using the faucet to make bottles for their infants. A health worker I spoke to kept a Crock-pot in her bathroom that she filled with bottled water, heated, and then poured into the tub for bathing.

It took too long to come, but in time the nation took notice of what happened in this American city. An unusually bright spotlight shined on the Flint Water Crisis not only because its story is an unusually painful one of compromised water and disenfranchised residents, but because it made intersecting systems of power visible. Indeed, the water crisis can be understood as a public health story, an economic story, a political story, and an environmental story. It can be understood in terms of infrastructure, systemic racism, inequality, medicine, activism, money, public policy, journalism, sociology, urbanism, complex systems, and science. It is a story of families and children, of education, of institutions, and of history.

All these stories are factual, but it is in their intersectionality that we can best see the truth.

What I appreciate about *Managing Challenges for the Flint Water Crisis* is that, in form and content, it embraces multiplicity in its approach. Unruliness is as inherent to anthologies as it is to democracy—a tangle of voices, opinions, priorities, and stances. But in both forums, participants build something new from a common foundation. Here, contributors wrestle with the complexities of Flint's story with a discerning eye toward how to contextualize it in history, and what its implications are for communities all across the country. At heart, their goals are the same: to create the conditions in our communities where life, liberty, and the pursuit of happiness is possible.

The Flint Water Crisis is in the strange position of being partly in history and partly in the news. The spring day of the infamous water switch is falling ever further back in time. The segregation and austerity that contributed to the city's vulnerability goes back much farther.

At the same time, the full consequences of the water crisis have yet to be seen. How will this generation of children fare? How will wraparound recovery services work (or not work)? What is the future for Flint as a sustainable, thriving, healthy city? What are the long-term implications of shifting water policies, service contracts, and expectations for water affordability and safety? How will Flint's story change (or not change) our understanding of what it takes to interrupt a dysfunctional cycle of urban disinvestment and infrastructure inequality? Will Flint finally provoke our nation into making it a priority to totally remove lead, one of the world's best known neurotoxins, from our drinking water system? Will any individual or entity ever be held legally accountable for choices that caused or prolonged the disaster? Who has the right to say that the Flint Water Crisis is "over"?

In both iterations, as history and as news, Flint's story still needs our attention, especially when it is traced out ecologically, which is to say, as one part of a whole—a life force within a connective civic system of cause-and-effect that stretches across time and space. To dig deep into this one community in Michigan is to better understand all communities. And the more people coming to the table to do the work, the better.

As I write this introduction, our world is deep in the coronavirus pandemic. In just a few months, more Americans have died from COVID-19 than those who died in the wars in Vietnam, Afghanistan, and Iraq, *combined*— though some regions and communities experienced an especially large share of the suffering. While healthcare leaders and frontline workers navigate the most urgent demands of the virus, tensions are escalating about how to manage quarantines, states-of-emergency, and political leadership.

It is difficult to imagine, then, a more worthwhile time to consider the ways that we might best fuse the wisdom of communities of practice, resident stakeholders, and scholarship to navigate disasters that threaten public health, as the editors of this volume set out to do. May those who make a study of this take to heart the common-good ideals that are the implicit foundation of any community, and all the more necessary to guide us in times of crisis.

CHAPTER 1

IMPLICATIONS OF SOCIAL MEDIA ON DISASTER RESPONSE: COMMENTARY ON THE FLINT TWITTERVERSE

Gina Rico Mendez, Megan Stubbs-Richardson,
Somya Mohanty and Arthur G. Cosby

Introduction

The Flint water crisis is a profound humanitarian disaster for the citizens of Flint, Michigan. It is also an event that has captured the attention of individuals throughout the United States and indeed the world through extensive media coverage. It is unthinkable to many that a developed country can have a city whose water supply is poisoning its citizens, and that the government failed to respond in an appropriate, timely manner to the water contamination. Given the increasing use of internet-based communication, this technological crisis created a high volume of human communication in the digital news and social media. It is apparent that humans are using social media as a new form of adaptation for dealing with extreme events and its challenges such as the Flint water crisis.[1]

This chapter will explore the possibilities and pitfalls of online communication during critical events by discussing the collective ability of social media users to communicate, reach out to others for collective action, and organize in response to the negative consequences of the Flint disaster through the lens of Twitter. Rather than focusing on the technical aspects of data collection and analysis, a wide variety of audiences can be reached with key messages through social media, which has the capacity to transform the way public and private sectors and civil society manage critical events in general (and technological disasters in particular). The chapter begins by describing the event as observed on the Twitter platform, followed by some inferences from the data that build on existing theoretical and empirical work about social media and disasters.

Flint's Twitterverse

Twitter is a widely used microblogging platform that allows users to post brief (formerly a 140-character limit, changing to a 280-character limit in

November 2017) messages known as "tweets" and interact with others through following, likes, and re-tweets. Each day, there are about a half billion tweets generated worldwide from over 310 million users.[2] Across all social media platforms, Twitter is used most often for reading and discussing the news, therefore, it is proven to be a highly "event driven" media platform that can be used to learn about individual and collective attitudes and behavior.[3] Twitter was developed in the United States and has a heavy social media footprint throughout the country. For these reasons, this platform is considered a very useful resource for investigating human response to high profile events in the United States, such as the Flint water crisis.

The Flint water crisis clearly became a high-profile event when the state of Michigan declared it the Flint Water Crisis to constitute "a state of emergency" in early January 2016. With this announcement, media attention focusing on the lead contamination in the Flint water system, including social media activity, began to increase. Over the next several weeks, many significant events occurred that helped structure a timeline for the digital Flint Twitterverse:

- The state of Michigan declared a state of emergency for Flint on the same day that the Environmental Protection Agency announced a federal investigation into the matter (January 5, 2016).

- Michael Moore, filmmaker and activist who is also a resident of Flint, expanded his webpage to include a petition to arrest Michigan Governor Snyder for his role in the Flint Crisis[4] because he felt it was not being adequately covered by traditional media (January 6, 2016).

- President Obama issued a statement declaring Flint to be a federal emergency area and made available 5 million dollars in federal funds (January 16, 2016).

- Presidential candidates weighed in on this crisis (e.g., Bernie Sanders on January 16 and Hillary Clinton on January 17 of 2016).

- Michigan governor Rick Snyder delivered the State of the State address to the legislature that included both a call for $28 million in funding for Flint and an apology: "I am sorry, and I will fix it" (January 19, 2016).

- *Time Magazine* published an influential article overviewing the Flint Crisis, entitled "The Toxic Tap" (February 1, 2016).

During January and February of 2016, Twitter activity addressing the Flint Crisis began to rapidly increase. In these two months, the full firehose of archived tweets provided by the social media aggregation company Gnip[5] yielded about 2.5 million tweets discussing the Flint water crisis. These tweets were generated by approximately 80,000 different Twitter accounts. This estimate of Twitter activity on Flint was obtained by filtering the firehose of tweets using the following keywords and hashtags:

> *Flint water, Flint lead poisoning, Flint water poisoning, Flint volunteer, Flint volunteering, Flint aid, Flint help, #Flint, #FlintWater, #FlintWaterCrisis, #FlintHelp, #HelpFlint, #FlintLivesMatter, #FlintOp, and #NewPipesForFlint.*

Tweets using these keywords and hashtags were collected globally from January 3, 2016 to February 28, 2016.

If additional keywords and hashtags were applied, it is likely that more tweets would be identified, suggesting that this two-month Twitterverse would be even larger than 2.5 million tweets.

Figure 1 provides a depiction of the daily Twitter traffic for January and February of 2016. There are several patterns that are worth noting. First, there was a comparably low level of Twitter activity at the beginning of 2016. However, an examination of the content of these tweets indicates that users at this stage were focusing on the severity of the water poisoning, the health risks, especially for children, and the accountability of government officials. Second, even though the announcement of a state of emergency and an investigation being launched by the EPA occurred on January 5th, the rapid expansion of the Flint Crisis Twitterverse did not take off until about a week later on January 13th. Given the content and users that produced the tweets, this increase is attributed to the focus on the topic among presidential candidates from the Democratic party. During the next week, there was an extremely rapid growth of Twitter activity, which peaked on January 21st, a few days after President Obama's declaration of Flint as a federal emergency, Governor Snyder's State of the State address apologizing for the crisis, and comments from presidential candidates Sanders and Clinton. There was another smaller but significant spike in the frequency of Twitter messages at the beginning of February that coincided with the Toxic Tap article in *Time Magazine*. During the rest of February, there were modest spikes, but an overall clear decline and leveling of the size of the Flint Twitterverse.

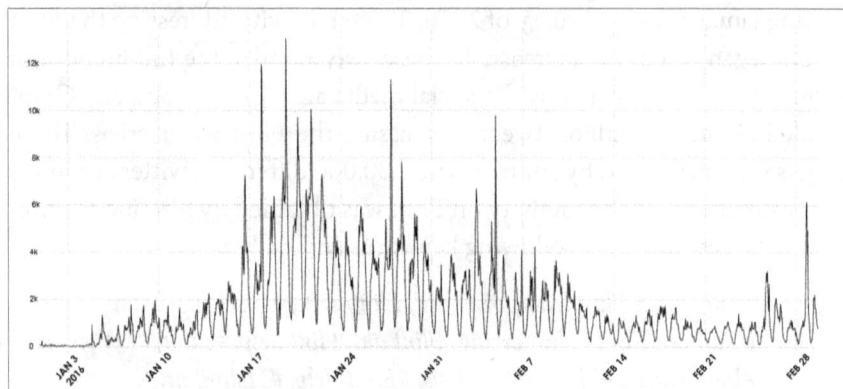

Figure 1. Daily Data Volume

Understanding Twitter During Extreme Events

Twitter data provides an important lens through which to understand the nature of social media discussions during an extreme event. It also allows for analysis of the form and strength of networks that develop around important issues, and organic or self-organizing behavior as a response or adaptation to a crisis. There is gathering evidence that social media can encourage and enable organic and self-organizing responses to extreme situations such as natural disasters, technological disasters, or terrorist events.[6] In the realm of collective action facing these types of critical events, social media has the potential to enhance rapid response and resilience.[7] By reviewing social media activity during several recent extreme events, it is possible to identify important patterns of behavior and communication. The study of the Flint water crisis in Twitter evidence supports these patterns.

It is common to find cases of social media usage to promote community-based responses during natural disasters such as Hurricane Sandy, the 2011 Tōhoku earthquake and tsunami, or the 2013 Pakistani Earthquake, when social media became an important aspect of disaster response and community resilience.[8] For example, during Hurricane Sandy, Twitter was extensively used to request and offer assistance and organize groups to aid others impacted by the disaster.[9] This organic or self-organizing behavior utilizing social media may very well represent a new form of resilience during extreme events. In similar fashion, "big data" enterprises such as the ride sharing company Uber are emerging as important self-organizing forces during emergency situations. Uber was utilized during the 2015 Paris terrorist incident to evacuate individuals from the site of the attack.[10] An even more adaptive example is the recent Indian based Uber-like service Ola, which responded to the flooding in India by rapidly including boats as a service to evacuate people during the flooding.[11]

However, responses from social media users may differ in cases of technological disasters, such as the Flint water crisis. For Baum et al. (1983, 334-5), technological catastrophes are human made events such as "accidents, failures, or mishaps involving the technology and manipulation of the natural environment that we have created to support our standard of living." During these situations, victims experience further uncertainties of personal and social consequences of the disaster. Many are seeking compensation or searching for who is accountable for the catastrophe, which can lead to conflicts between citizens, public organizations or businesses, government entities, and politicians. In addition, as social capital in communities affected by technological disasters tends to be fragile, the internal recovery initiatives are often minimal and open the door for outsiders to lead these efforts (RCAC 2004).

Social media could potentially facilitate outsider recovery efforts by reducing coordination and communication costs and eliminating problems of physical distance. It can also enhance victims' reactions as they seek help and/or investigate and publicize the anomalies that led to the disaster. In the case of Flint, there were abundant responses from outsiders who promoted campaigns to collect funds for relief and send water to Flint. Inside the community of Flint, there is a widespread campaign to hold bureaucrats and politicians accountable for their actions and claims for social justice.

Observing the Twitterverse

To summarize the approximately 2.5 million tweets that were collected during the 2-month study, several social analytics were used to detect patterns of communication and networks within the Flint Twitterverse. These included examinations of trend data, time specific word clouds, Klout scores (social media influence scores), networks of Twitter users (network analysis), and networks of concepts (word collation analysis).[12] The results of these analyses were used to shape and inform the commentary in this chapter. Based on this initial investigation, three major themes of organic or self-organizing tweets were occurring in the Twitterverse. These were 1) organizing humanitarian responses, 2) government accountability and citizen's participation, and 3) social justice.

Organizing Humanitarian Responses

Several sub-categories of tweets can be discerned within the humanitarian theme: 1) self-organizing for help, 2) raising funds for Flint primarily through crowdsourcing, 3) recognizing organizations or groups for their efforts to help the people of Flint, and 4) challenging others to assist the citizens of Flint. This theme (Table 1) reveals how individuals used social media to organize disaster and relief efforts for victims of the Flint Water Crisis. Many of these efforts were organized by individuals, groups, local companies, celebrities, and larger corporations. Some tweets consisted of providing information via hyperlinks about how to help the people of Flint. Also, many tweets included websites with direct links to online crowdsourcing programs, such as GoFundMe and Beyonce's *#BeyGood* campaign. Other tweets suggested making disaster relief efforts a challenge. For example, one hashtag, *#GroceryStoreForFlint* challenges other companies, including Kroger and Walmart, by name to have a "race" in their assistance for Flint victims.

One aspect of these tweets that is particularly interesting is the fact that "who" is organizing outreach efforts is often mentioned. This could possibly be an attempt to motivate others to get more involved in assisting the people of Flint. These tweets tend to provide credit to volunteerism by recognizing the individual and/or collective efforts of organized behavior. Further, many different individuals and companies of diverse backgrounds and locations tweeted their interest in organizing large outreach efforts for Flint, such as VanDrie (a Michigan-based furniture company). There are numerous other examples of tweets that recognize organizations and groups to assist in the Flint efforts, such as Michigan State University organizing students to help Flint, inmates in an Ionia, MI prison pledging one-third of their monthly income to support bottled water donations, and a Michigan-based Muslim humanitarian organization collecting and distributing bottled water.

Government Accountability and Citizen Participation

Research on disasters often make a distinction between natural disasters and technological disasters. As mentioned earlier, this distinction can have profound implications on the nature of human response, reaction, and the interpretations of events. At the very center of this distinction is the commonly held view that natural disasters such as hurricanes, tornadoes, and

Table 1. Humanitarian Tweets: Examples from
the Flint Water Crisis Twitterverse

For those who are looking for ways to help #Flint, here's some info for you. Please share. #FlintWaterCrisis https://t.co/JCTBnXbD4o

---

HELP: All VanDrie locations are collecting bottled drinking water through Friday to deliver to #Flint! More info: https://t.co/XaH4jEGbee

---

RT: Beyoncé Announces #BeyGood Campaign to Aid Children Affected by Flint Water Crisis https://t.co/FZwG1hJnNqhttps://t.co/46QlTGCEdc

---

RT #GroceryStoreForFlint Let's make it a race! First one wins! @meijer @Walmart @kroger @SaveALot Help them! #FlintTownHall #Flin...

RT @ComplexMusic: Salute @MeekMill for contributing to the Flint Water Crisis relief in a big way: https://t.co/qCWiRK0v3v https://t.co/DIi...

---

https://t.co/jaU0x80DPq Beyonce Joins Diddy, Mark Wahlberg and Big Sean to Aid Relief Efforts for Flint Water Cri... https://t.co/L8w625un0P

RT Muslim Charity @LIFEforRELIEF dist. 100K+ water bottles, volunteers walking nghborhds in major relief effort. #FlintWaterCrisi...

RT Wanna help out the victims of the #FlintWaterCrisis? Donate https://t.co/ltN2GhCatW

RT @essencemag: Big Sean launches #HealFlintKids fundraiser to help during #FlintWaterCrisis: https://t.co/CtqusLYTtc https://t.co/Dz0sNYoU...

@NSBE Launches #GoFundMe Campaign to Help Flint. Donate now: https://t.co/QQlbGezcJT Setting up a Gofundme for #FlintWaterCrisis need everyone help!!

RT MSULiveOn: Spartans! Head to student services tomorrow to discover ways to help Flint through the water crisis #SpartansWill...

#Michigan prisoners pledge to donate a third of their monthly incomes to help #Flint https://t.co/sxXEG7Qrfd

---

earthquakes are acts of nature, and consequently humans or human organizations do not cause or produce the core disaster. But technological disasters such as oil spills, train wrecks, nuclear power plant failures, and toxic waste spills are typically seen as caused by human failures or neglect. The Flint water crisis can be classified as a disaster of the second type, and the Flint Twitterverse is replete with examples of messages calling for accountability and pointing to individuals and organizations that were responsible for the lead exposure to the citizens of Flint.

The Flint crisis also had another dimension that influenced the high level of accountability discussion. Flint is home to the highly influential activist and film producer Michael Moore. He was recognized by *Time Magazine* in 2005 as one of the world's 100 Most Influential People.[13] Michael Moore's entry into the Flint crisis has primarily been one of promoting his view of accountability and responsibility for governmental failure. He has focused his attention on Governor Rick Snyder and his administration. On his website, he promotes the hashtag *#ArrestGovernorSnyder*, and has an ongoing petition for Governor Snyder to resign and be arrested by the Federal Bureau of Investigation (FBI). By mid-May, Moore's website reports that over 600,000 individuals have signed the Snyder petition. There is little doubt that Moore's media activism, including that on Twitter, has helped shape the discussions of the Flint water crisis.

One of the likely outcomes of technological disasters is engagement in blaming narratives. As can be seen in Table 2, this is also true for the Flint water crisis. Within this theme, several narratives of blaming appear, including: 1) holding Governor Snyder accountable by responding to the petition that Michael Moore put together using *#ArrestGovernorSnyder*, 2) blaming arguments that shift back and forth between elected Republicans and Democrats, and 3) a general discussion of blame generated at politicians and the government's role in the Flint water crisis. Most tweets tended to focus either on blaming Governor Snyder or signing the Michael Moore petition for his resignation and incarceration.

Table 2. Accountability Tweets: Examples from
   the Flint Water Crisis Twitterverse

So important to set precedent in holding Gov. Snyder accountable 4 #Flint. Other city/state officials can learn.

Rep Lawrence: Emergency Manager Act dissolves home rule; therefore, local govt (Flint) should not be held responsible. #FlintWaterCrisis

Hold the gov accountable for poisoning Flint. Sign the petition: https://t.co/FyneHya82e@moveon #FlintWaterCrisis #ArrestGovSnyder

RT @Usher: I signed a petition to help hold Gov. Synder accountable for poisoning Flint children. Will you? https://t.co/HJNm4CPsKx

Governor Knew About Flint Water Poisoning for Nearly a Year, Tried to Shift Blame https://t.co/ZMDOLnUpvb

RT @Eclectablog: Why is the man most to blame for the #FlintWaterCrisis still the Emergency Manager of Detroit schools? https://t.co/CGw8md...

RT @starfirst: Republicans Laughably Try to Blame Democrats For Flint Water Poisoning https://t.co/DO5qfPBqOB via @politicususa

Dems caused POLLUTED H2O in Flint why blame GOV as sole source problem. Look to the Mayor who started the issue https://t.co/uaKg4X4anZ

Michigan governor: solve Flint water crisis instead of laying blamehttps://t.co/2siy1IAnGV

Republicans pointing finger at EPA instead of #Flint Governor, really says how can we blame PBO. #FlintWaterCrisis

Instead of bitching about blame, fix the #FlintWaterCrisis already. It's going on 2 years now. Worry about fault later.

Emergency manager told flint to stop buying detroit water? to tie into Flint River? Nope. blame flint politicians https://t.co/aDEyodgjQY

SNYDER IS NOT TO BLAME. The lead in the water is the fault of the local government, NOT THE GOVERNOR #DemDebate #FlintWaterCrisis

RT: While he poisoned children, GovSnyder gave clean water to GM plant #Flintwater corroded their parts. Unbelievably evil and...

RT: Somewhere a kid is in jail over a dime bag of weed. But no one is behind bars for poisoning an entire city of children. #Fl...

RT: Sanders: "I did ask for the resignation of Gov. Snyder. His irresponsibility was so outrageous." #FlintWaterCrisis #DemDebate

Social Justice

Flint is one of the America's poorest large cities and has been experiencing a long-term trend of economic decline—the average median household income in Flint is $24,679 compared to the American average of $53,482, while the percentage of persons in poverty is 41.6% versus the national average of 14.6%. The city has consistently lost population over the last several decades as automotive industry jobs have left the area. Accompanying this period of economic distress, the city's racial composition has also changed from a majority white community to a majority African American community. The reality that the poisoning of the drinking water occurred in a predominantly African American community raises questions about race and racism as factors in the creation of the problem and in the response (or lack thereof) to the crisis. Dialogue about race and racism emerged as one of the important themes in the Flint Twitterverse.

The Flint Twitterverse includes numerous accusations and interpretations of the crisis having roots in race and racism (Table 3). The dialogue also includes numerous counter arguments maintaining that race was not a factor, or that "the race card" was being used. Michael Moore's accusation of "racial genocide" and Hillary Clinton's tweet, "would it have happened if they were rich and white instead of poor and black?" are examples of high-profile interpretations of the crisis as a form of racism. Interestingly, adjectives describing racism included not only genocide, but also references to environmental racism and structural racism. Counter arguments were occasionally in direct reaction to accusations of racism. For example, Governor Snyder stated that race had no role in the response to the Flint water crisis. The subcategories identified under this theme include the following: 1) providing information to build the argument that the crisis response was due to racism, classism, or the intersection of the two, 2) arguing that certain groups would consistently make unrelated issues about race, and 3) arguing that race had no role in the Flint water crisis.

Table 3. Social Justice Tweets: Examples from
the Flint Water Crisis Twitterverse

RT @markmobility: #FlintWaterCrisis - 99,000 residents - 57% Black - 40% Poor - 9,000 kids with lead poisoning Flint HOSPITAL Water: https...

RT @markmobility: #FlintWaterCrisis - 99,000 residents - 57% Black - 40% Poor - 9,000 kids with lead poisoning Flint HOSPITAL Water: https...

RT @larryelder: Democrats And The Race Card: Don't Leave Home Without It #FlintWaterCrisis #DemDebate https://t.co/AQdrSpfMV4

Race baiting. The switch in water supply was cost saving measure. Wouldn't happen in a rich black community either. https://t.co/9d9UHn26Av

RT @AP: Flint, Mich., asks what role race, wealth and class have played in public health crisis caused by lead in water: https://t.co/YQyNs...

Michigan Governor Says Race Had No Role in Flint Water Response https://t.co/bBtETfyOPP

RT: The potential long-term damage caused by the lead poisoning of children in Flint, Michigan should Outrage ALL OF US Regardless of race!

RT @billmckibben: MI Gov who says 'race played no role' in #flintwatercrisis is simply lying. No possible chance this would have happened i...

RT @RestingPlatypus: Race Is in the Air We Breathe and the Water We Drink: The Moral Failure in 9.Flint @HuffPostBloghttps://t.co/kGSwidE5cg...

RT @DorothyERoberts: #Race is not an innate biological category, but #racism has deadly biological effects. #FlintWaterCrisis #FatalInventi...

RT @MSNBC: EXCLUSIVE: @HillaryClinton writes about race, justice & the #FlintWaterCrisis in MSNBC op-ed https://t.co/ln0TunPzA7https://t.c...

RT @CharlesMBlow: Clinton bringing up the #FlintWaterCrisis. This is an outrageous story. Google it... #PoisionWater #Race #DemDebate

Flint's structural racism: This is why providing poisoned water to the city's citizens seemed like a reasonable idea https://t.co/BFNPLnCSyX

'Racism' Behind Flint Water Crisis – But Majority-Black City Council Started It Allhttps://t.co/5b4yCQR6ws

Environmental racism Flint, Michigan: Did race and poverty factor into water crisis? @CNN https://t.co/DLGVoCZyEL

Michael Moore determines that the Flint water crisis is racist genocide https://t.co/UoBZFkmxBJ

The Racist Roots Of Flint's Water Crisis https://t.co/ LWSA1CIqWC#BlackLivesMatter #OscarsSoWhite #Racism #Assault #Crime

The #FlintWaterCrisis is the most egregious case of environmental racism/classism in my lifetime. On par w/ #Tuskegee and #JimCrow or worse. RT @HuffPostPol:

Conclusion

It is evident that the Flint Twitterverse created novel forms of human adaptation, organization, and response to the Flint water crisis in ways that could not have occurred prior to the advent of social media. In fact, Twitter was being used to create virtual communities that were capable of expanding conversation about the crisis, and producing actions that were having impact on the humanitarian response, public accountability, and collective interpretations of the crisis. Significantly, Twitter users were promoting a mode of social organization that was both self-organized and independent from traditional hierarchical schemes of authority. Additionally, the very nature of Internet-based interaction was producing outcomes that were either eliminating or reducing the restraining effects of physical distance to promoting collective actions. In the Flint data, there were abundant responses from outsiders who promoted campaigns to collect funds for relief and send water to Flint. Both inside and outside the community of Flint, there was a wide-spread and intense campaign to hold bureaucrats and politicians accountable for their actions, as well as to promote calls for social justice.

Flint is an example of how social media platforms such as Twitter can be used to engage citizens in public affairs debates. In some respects, the Flint data depicts Twitter as a forum for both the participation of the disenfranchised and less powerful in an important public issue, as well as that for the more powerful and elite members of society to show support for these issues. In general, there are optimistic views suggesting that the Internet promotes access to information and allows open participation in online debates. However, there are other perspectives suggesting that online interactions are likely to follow the same patterns of the political world and issues, such as information bias, lack of access, and power structures in which elites define content and in general Internet literacy. The Flint Twitterverse is highly complex and there is ample evidence to support both of these seemingly opposing perspectives. There are numerous examples of elites and the powerful utilizing Twitter to promote their views on humanitarian approaches to the crisis, accountability and responsibility, and social justice. At the same time, the data is replete with examples of "everyday citizens" tweeting their views on the same topics. Both perspectives have valid points and are not mutually exclusive.

The Flint Twitterverse provided an opportunity to examine the role of social media amid a technological disaster and provides insight into the relationship between democracy and the Internet. In this regard, the Twitter activity around the Flint water crisis created the conditions that enabled deliberation and enhanced democratic debate. This is the result of increased access and ease of the spread of information, reduction of the complexities of face-to-face interaction, and the provision of an open forum to express the opinions in public debates.[14] Dalberg suggests that in a deliberative model of Internet democracy rhetoric and practice that there is potential to create and expand an inclusive public sphere by fostering rational public opinion which enhances accountability.[15] This may have special implications for technological disasters because it enables citizens to address not only the negative effects of the disaster but also the distrust and dissatisfaction with the government. In the Flint crisis, Twitter allowed citizens to create online communities, spread information, and engage with others to report the salient aspects of the crisis and to promote accountability.

Notes

1.   Bernabé-Moreno, J., A. Tejeda-Lorente, C. Porcel, and E. Herrera-Viedma. "Leveraging Localized Social Media Insights for Early Warning Systems." *Procedia Computer Science* 31 (2014): 1051–60; Hossmann, Theus, Paolo Carta, Dominik Schatzmann, Franck Legendre, Per Gunningberg, and Christian Rohner. "Twitter in Disaster Mode: Security Architecture." *Architecture.* SWID '11 Proceedings of the Special Workshop on Internet and Disasters, Article No. 7 (2011); Saleem, Haji Mohammad, Yishi Xu and Derek Ruths. "Novel Situational Information in Mass Emergencies: What Does Twitter Provide?" *Procedia Engineering* 78 (2014): 155–164.

2.   DMR. By the Numbers: 170+ Amazing Twitter Statistics. 2016. http://expan

dedramblings.com/index.php/march-2013-by-the-numbers-a-few-amazing-twitter-stats/ (accessed May 21, 2016).

3. Murthy, Dhiraj. "Towards a Sociological Understanding of Social Media: Theorizing Twitter." *Sociology* 46 no 6 (2012):1059–73.

4. http://michaelmoore.com/ArrestGovSnyder/

5. Paid service provided by Twitter that pushes data to end users in near real-time, and guarantees delivery of 100% of the tweets that match the search criteria.

6. Centers for Disease Control and Prevention. Crisis and Emergency Risk Communication 2014 ed. U.S. Department of Health and Human Services: 2014. Retrieved from https://emergency.cdc.gov/cerc/resources/pdf/cerc_2014edition.pdf; Hossmann, et al. "Twitter in Disaster Mode: Security Architecture." *Architecture.* SWID '11 Proceedings of the Special Workshop on Internet and Disasters, Article No. 7 (2011); Magsino, Sammantha L. (Ed.). Applications of Social Network Analysis for Building Community Disaster Resilience. Workshop Summary. Washington, D.C.: The National Academy Press (2009). Retrieved from https://www.nap.edu/download/12706

7. Colander, David, and Roland Kupers. *Complexity and the Art of Public Policy: Solving Society's Problems from the Bottom Up.* Princeton, N.J.: Princeton University Press, 2014.

8. Keim, Mark E., and Eric Noji. "Emergent Use of Social Media: A New Age of Opportunity for Disaster Resilience." *American Journal of Disaster Medicine* 6, no 1 (2011): 47–54; Kongthon, Alisa, Choochart Haruechaiyasak, and Jaruwat Pailai. "The Role of Twitter during a Natural Disaster: Case Study of 2011 Thai Flood." Proceedings of PICMET '12: Technology Management for Emerging Technologies. (2012): 2227–32; Landwehr, Peter M., and Kathleen M. Carley. *Social Media in Disaster Relief. In Data Mining and Knowledge Discovery for Big Data. Studies in Big Data 1.* Edited by Wesley W. Chu. Berlin, Heidelberg: Springer (2014).

9. Edwards, John F., Somya Mohanty, and Patrick Fitzpatrick. Assessment of Social Media Usage During Sever Weather Events and the Development of a Twitter-based Model for Improved Communication of Storm-related Information. Starkville, MS (2015): Coastal Storm Awareness Program, NOAA.

10. Hawkins, Andrew J. "Tracing the Spread of Uber Rumors during the Paris Terrorist Attacks." *The Verge,* November 16 (2015): http://www.theverge.com/2015/11/16/9745782/uber-paris-terrorism-rumors-twitter-facebook (accessed April 22, 2016).

11. The Times of India. "Ola Launches Boat Service in Flood-Affected Chennai." *The Times of India* (2015). http://timesofindia.indiatimes.com/tech/tech-news/

Ola-launches-boat-service-in-flood-affected-Chennai/articleshow/49816195.
cms (Accessed May 22, 2016).

12. Schaefer, Mark. *Return on Influence: The Revolutionary Power of Klout, Social Scoring, and Influence Marketing.* New York, NY (2012): McGraw-Hill; Rao, Adithya, Nemanja Spasojevic, Zhisheng Li, and Trevor D Souza. "Klout Score: Measuring Influence Across Multiple Social Networks." IEEE International Big Data Conference - Workshop on Mining Big Data in Social Networks (2005): http://arxiv.org/pdf/1510.08487v1.pdf (Accessed April 20, 2016).

13. Penn, Sean. "Michael Moore." *Time Magazine* 165 no 16 (2005): http://content.time.com/time/specials/packages/article/0,28804,1972656_197269 6_1973072,00.html (Accessed May 22, 2016).

14. Papacharissi, Zizi. "The Virtual Sphere: The Internet as a Public Sphere." *New Media and Society* 4, no 1 (2002): 9–27.

15. Dahlberg, Lincoln. "The Internet, Deliberative Democracy, and Power: Radicalizing the Public Sphere." *International Journal of Media and Cultural Politics* 3, no 1 (2007): 47–64.

CHAPTER 2

BROKEN PROMISES IN THE VEHICLE CITY: FLINT'S CRISIS OF DISTRUST

Megan Ruxton

Introduction

The water crisis that erupted in Flint, Michigan has gained national attention from the media, politicians, and celebrities alike. This most recent blow to the city's population is a symptom of another crisis, one beginning nearly a century ago, that has evolved and grown to staggering proportions. Manifesting in far less obvious forms, the city of Flint suffers from a crisis of self, a crisis of identity, and above all, a crisis of distrust. After decades of declining conditions, residents of this Rustbelt city have persevered in the face of economic hardship, staggering rates of unemployment, a crumbling infrastructure, and now, debilitating illness and disease as the result of public policy made in the absence of democratic representation. The City of Flint stood its ground, time and again attempting to revitalize and renew; however, the most recent breach of trust between the people and those who are supposed to govern them has shaken the faith of even the most ardent optimists.

On January 5, 2016, Michigan Governor Rick Snyder declared a state of emergency for Flint due to dangerously high levels of lead in the drinking water.[1] Local media has documented the situation since April 2014, when the city switched from the Detroit water system to the Flint River as a cost-saving measure. Following this switch, residents complained of drinking water that was discolored, foul-smelling, and unfit for consumption—complaints that were not taken seriously until months later when Governor Snyder was forced to take action.[2] As the national spotlight concentrated on the poverty-stricken, majority African American city, failures at all levels of government came to light. As coverage of the Flint water crisis continues, a major element of the media narrative has been and continues to be the distrust of political and government leaders fostered amongst the citizens of Flint. The revelation that the water crisis was caused by the same government officials who had dismissed residents' concerns for nearly two years, has been suggested as the death knell for the relationship of trust between citizens of Flint and their government.

The argument set forth here is that the death knell tolled long ago; this most recent breach of trust was simply the final nail in the coffin. This chapter discusses the Flint water crisis as the capstone to decades of declining relationships between Flint citizens and their local and state governments. The situation in Flint, a city that is mostly African American with a high proportion of families in poverty, has evoked particular concern about environmental justice and racial inequality. The consequences of this broken relationship entail normative and practical implications for the residents of Flint, and government officials from City Hall to the Governor's mansion. Flint is not alone and could be any one of the many American cities struggling to survive following deindustrialization. For Flint and other cities like it, the road to Hell has been paved with good intentions; however, these good intentions have been supplemented with racist and classist housing practices, business-friendly policies, and most recently, a laundry list of government agencies and officials acting with "intransigence, unpreparedness, delay, [and] inaction."[3] The following pages will examine how these practices have led to the current water crisis, how they have contributed to the lack of trust that has gripped Flint, and what can be expected as the citizens of Flint attempt to persevere in the latest of a series of setbacks for the once-booming Vehicle City.

Political Trust in Theory and Practice

Political trust has been an issue of concern in the field of political science and public administration for decades. America in the early 1960s was still a nation of optimism regarding government. In his highly influential article on the relevance of political trust, Hetherington quotes Lane's 1962 work on political ideology: "If they think of the government as affecting their lives at all, [they] think of it as giving benefits and protections."[4] Hetherington uses this to introduce the change that has occurred in the decades since, with a nearly uninterrupted downward slide for political trust in the United States and a public that no longer thinks warmly of government as "giving benefits and protections," but instead as "producing scandal, waste, and unacceptable intrusions on people's personal lives."[5] Since Lane's piece, however, debate has raged over what trust really is, how it is measured (and what that represents), and what the causes and consequences of a lack of trust may be.

Generalized trust can be understood as a mental construct, a relationship between one individual and another individual, group, or institution. Trust is an association, an assumed vulnerability on the part of an individual with the belief that another party would not harm or betray him or her despite being capable of doing so. This assumption is conditional, an iterative calculation based on the perceptions of actions taken by the other party. Political trust, then, is an evaluative judgment toward government based on the normative expectations individuals have on how the government should or should not be acting.[6] Trust can be understood as specific or diffuse, the former being evaluations of incumbents within the institutions, and the latter being evaluations of the institutions themselves.[7] While most would agree that political trust is a necessary component of a functioning democracy, there is disagreement among scholars on several of the finer points: how much trust is required, and whether or not a certain amount of distrust—or skepticism—is a normal, healthy part of a democratic system of checks and balances.[8]

Political trust in the United States, among all demographics and at a mostly constant rate, has declined to an all-time low since the trust-in-government questions were first included in the American National Election Studies survey in the early 1960s. These declining levels of trust at the federal level occur for a number of reasons. Incumbent evaluations do play a large part, particularly presidential performance in terms of economics, as well as the personal qualities of the president. In addition, evaluations are influenced by whether the president is of the same party as the survey respondent, as well as satisfaction with the policies being promoted by those in government.[9] Dissatisfaction with political parties, by ideological extremists or more centrist voters, also appears to be correlated with expressions of distrust in government.[10] Levi and Stoker summarize a large mass of previous work on political trust showing several additional factors for declining trust in the U.S.—political scandals, critical media messages about government, public perceptions of unsolved problems such as crime and family decline, increasing dissatisfaction with Congress, and an increasingly frequent perception that politicians overall acted selfishly and were unresponsive to constituents.[11]

Both specific and diffuse support are interwoven into the larger concept of political trust, with each dimension influencing and influenced by the other. The consequences of this for governance are concerning; as trust diminishes, incumbent approval is diminished, which in turn undermines the ability of these incumbents to attempt to solve problems, which itself further diminishes trust and incumbent approval. Without an exogenous shock to the system, this cycle continues indefinitely.[12] While economic and incumbent performance can have positive influences on trust, the effects appear to be short-term and asymmetrical: a strong economy does little to increase trust, while a very poor economy can have a strong impact on the loss of trust.[13] Normatively, this is troubling: "More trust translates into warmer feelings for [elected officials and political institutions], which in turn provides leaders more leeway to govern effectively and institutions a larger store of support regardless of the performance of those running the government."[14] A lack of trust sets the public at odds with those whose actions will be under constant scrutiny and vulnerable to possible electoral repercussion. Government officials making difficult decisions—for good or ill will be criticized harshly and could face a lack of compliance and potentially widespread discontent and protest.[15]

While the finer points of political trust at the federal level can be used to answer questions regarding the public-governmental relationship, the United States is a diverse and multifaceted nation. When aggregating at the federal level, variation between localities is masked, this oversight prompted Rahn and Rudolph[16] to examine municipalities and examine why political trust is higher in some areas than in others. This is vital for several reasons: local governments have independent authority to make policy decisions ranging from taxes to education to environmental regulation; they have been given a high degree of authority and responsibility through federal devolution of power; and there is also evidence that local political trust and national political trust are independent from one another.[17] Rahn and Rudolph's integrated model indicates that local political trust is the product of both individual and city-level factors. Of particular interest, they found that individuals' racial identity and perception of their own political efficacy, as well as their perception of local conditions, were significant factors in levels of trust. Representational systems, on the other hand, and the performance of political institutions were strong predictors for the city-level variables. In general, African Americans expressed lower levels of trust, a trend found at the national level as well. However, while this finding has been confirmed at the local level, Rahn and Rudolph's results "also suggest that the magnitude of such racial disparities in political trust is moderated by political representation."[18] In other words, when African Americans feel they have a voice in government—whether through ward-level elections that provide more representation for majority-minority districts or through African Americans in elected office—trust in local government is higher. When that representation is removed, there is a lack of belief in political efficacy, and the local system appears unresponsive and ineffective, levels of trust appear quite low.

This supports the findings of a large body of research on human behavior states that "citizens question their relationship with government and experience disenfranchisement when the following conditions are present: 1) citizens believe that local government is using its power against them or otherwise not helping them; 2) citizens do not feel part of local government, or they feel misunderstood or ignored; and 3) citizens find local government services and policies to be ineffective."[19] African Americans are the most likely to question the intentions and actions of local government, particularly regarding environmental health risks, partially as a result of feelings of increased vulnerability,[20] and partially as the result of institutional patterns of racial discrimination.

Racial disparities in trust in government is not isolated to elected officials; however, according to Stivers,[21] public administration has largely ignored the issue of race, despite its role as a "tragic harbinger" that shapes administrative decision-making in both theory and practice.[22] She argues that while individual public administrators are not necessarily themselves racist, administrative laws and management have been shaped by race-based policies of the Jim Crow era, which are no longer legally codified but have structured contemporary decisions. The discretion of street-level bureaucrats cannot be completely removed from the structures that have developed over decades of rules and regulations, which constrain and direct bureaucrats and can lead them to judge citizens as worthy of extraordinary help, worthy only of what the rules say and no more, or not worthy of help at all.[23] The combination of policies with race-based roots and individual bureaucratic discretion can result in the most vulnerable citizens feeling the most disenfranchised, forgotten, and ill-treated.

In the face of perceived mistreatment, these same vulnerable citizens are wary and distrustful of those who are supposed to be responsible for protecting them. Scammell, et al.[24] find that in the case of environmental health risks, vulnerable communities (those who feel the most powerless) are the least likely to trust those in authority, and are the most likely to question the motivations of those who are providing them with information. When government does attempt to address environmental health risks, if their information is at odds with the tangible evidence of citizens' own experiences, their information and remediation instructions may fall on deaf ears. When citizens lack trust in the source of any knowledge (i.e., a government agency), the validity of that knowledge is questioned. When the experiences of citizens are ignored by government officials, this feeds into the cycle of distrust, wherein citizens are dissatisfied with local conditions and the services provided, they believe their voices are not being heard or valued, and so the perception of government as a coercive tool of the powerful is reinforced, creating even more distrust.

Flint: A Crisis of Trust

"The Flint water crisis is a story of government failure, intransigence, unpreparedness, delay, inaction, and environmental injustice."[25] So begins the report of the Flint Water Advisory Task Force (FWATF), an independent advisory group tasked by Governor Snyder to review the actions that led to the Flint water crisis, and offer recommendations and guidelines for actions taken in the future.[26] As the opening line of the report indicates, failures at all levels of government are responsible for the current crisis, through purposeful action and inaction on the part of officials tasked with creating a safe and healthy water system. Countless news articles in 2016 indicated that the public's trust in government, particularly at the state and local level, has eroded to the point that some believe it will never recover. Emotional testimonies from Flint citizens have provided the backdrop to every report of increased lead in children's blood, the possibility of increased levels of miscarriages, deaths from Legionnaire's disease, and the overwhelming pile of evidence that officials knew of the risks months—even years—before informing the public of the hazards.[27]

While the water crisis is blamed for this erosion of trust, the citizens of Flint have been placed at a disadvantage, with circumstances chipping away at the relationship between citizens and government officials through a series of decisions over the last century. An overview of extant research on trust provides several factors that can help explain the lead-up to the current crisis, and the ensuing fallout. Trust is a continuum, and a dynamic one that resets with each new experience, and is the product of individual perception based on personal experience. Within local communities, distrust grows when personal efficacy and representation diminishes, when local conditions continue to decline, when policy promises are broken or are ineffectively implemented, and when government appears to empower the already powerful while ignoring those who are most in need. Each of these elements feeds into the cycle of distrust, so that when a crisis occurs, those most at risk are also those least likely to trust the information coming from those in authority, and so least likely to comply with the instructions they are being given. The story of Flint embodies this and can be used as a lens through which to view the modern American city.

A Foundation of Distrust

As Highsmith[28] argues, the city of Flint is not unique in its current dire straits. While the population reached a peak of 200,000 in 1960, today fewer than 100,000 citizens live within city limits; since 2000, 20 percent of the population has abandoned the city. As of 2014, 41.6 percent of the population lives below the federal poverty threshold, and 57 percent of the population is African American. The median value of owner-occupied housing is $36,700, only 20 percent of the national average.[29] Flint has its own unique history, connected indelibly to the rise and fall of the General Motors Company (GM). It shares many other qualities with other demographically similar cities facing alarmingly high rates of poverty, crime, unemployment, with the additional challenge of environmental risks at a disproportionate rate when compared to whiter, more affluent towns dotted across the country.[30]

Highsmith's narrative of the history of Flint examines how the once-booming company town has been forced into the position in which it now stands. Examining Flint's history through the lenses of legal, administrative, and popular segregation, as well as suburban versus metropolitan capitalism, Highsmith reveals a city caught in the forces of racially-based policies and free market idealism. Even as legal forms of racism have been eradicated, as Stivers[31] claims, the effects of those laws have shaped administrative management for decades afterwards. These discriminatory policies may continue to plague certain policy areas, particularly housing, where, beyond the practice of redlining, "the practice of denying or curtailing mortgage insurance, loans, and other goods and services based upon geographic, socioeconomic, and often racial considerations,"[32] is still pervasive. The segregationist policies preceding redlining had resulted in African Americans living in the least affluent areas of Flint, with lower-class whites faring only slightly better. Even after segregation was no longer codified, these areas were considered high-risk, and the assumption that racially and economically diverse neighborhoods lowered property values persisted. As a result, those who were able began to move to the suburbs where housing was more expensive, and higher taxes offered better schools and infrastructure.

GM had been a major employer for those living in the city, with manufacturing plants centrally located in Flint since 1903. Thousands of Flint residents relied on GM to provide steady employment and livable wages, especially the least affluent urban dwellers. The company sought to take advantage of the generous tax policies of the suburbs with new factories, while still ensuring they were accessible to their large workforce living in the city, many of them African American. To do so, GM encouraged and actively supported the attempts by the city of Flint to annex the outlying suburbs as part of its 1957-58 "New Flint" initiative, which would consolidate the city with its urbanized suburbs under a more efficient "super government" for the entire metropolitan area. This would provide shared tax revenue and the ability for municipal goods and services to be more evenly distributed and allow GM to better provide for its urban employees. The shared benefits would allow city employees to afford commuting to suburban plants, which would in turn increase the company's profits. The owners and managers of GM believed in the idea of metropolitan capitalism, which supported racial segregation, and favored suburbs over cities for development, but still wanted to maintain close ties to cities and their policymakers and residents.[33]

The New Flint initiative failed, as suburbs fought the attempts at annexation by incorporating, favoring the concept of suburban capitalism that focused on suburb-centered economic development alongside racial segregation as the means to ensure growth and prosperity. As the suburbs surrounding Flint chose to splinter into their own entities, Flint found itself constrained on all sides without additional room to encourage growth and began to watch its tax base and other income shrink. Additional efforts were made to entice businesses into the city with a series of tax abatements, of which GM and a few other manufacturers took advantage. However, without added tax revenue from the new businesses and with very few new jobs created (a provision which had not been included in the tax abatement plan), Flint still struggled to meet the needs of its vulnerable, shrinking population. Following the oil shocks of the 1970s, GM had to drastically restructure and reevaluate their strategy. It was at this point that company officials, "frustrated by their declining ability to control local politics and enticed by new opportunities overseas and in the states of the South and West, gave up on their metropolitan capitalist growth strategy and began disinvesting from the Flint area altogether."[34] Thousands of residents left to follow opportunities elsewhere, and those who stayed—whether because they wanted to or did not have the means to do otherwise—faced a dying city with few employment opportunities for low or unskilled urban residents. The final blow for Flint came in 1999 when GM closed its final facility, Buick City, and the plant that had once driven the area's economic engine was demolished, leaving an empty lot.[35]

City officials began to see economic problems in the form of budget shortfalls as early as the 1950s and 1960s, but these were only the beginning; over the years these occasional shortfalls translated into service cuts, municipal layoffs, rising service fees, delayed and sometimes deferred infrastructure maintenance, and ultimately the state's infamous imposition of an emergency manager for the city that many have argued was part of what has led to the most recent crisis.[36] Residents increasingly found themselves fighting for the basic needs of a community, while finding it more and more impossible to leave.

The shrinking and increasingly vulnerable population of Flint, mostly African American, with a large proportion of the citizens also struggling with poverty and unemployment, was already likely to be wary of government at all levels. As white residents with ample finances fled the area, the overwhelmingly African American residents who remained faced a local government still fighting a losing battle to convince businesses to stay and, in doing so, created additional financial burdens on residents in the form of higher fees, fewer and lower quality services, along with the daily challenges of life in a city that was literally crumbling beneath them. Promises to lure new business, jobs, and tourism resulted in aborted renewal projects and money spent on initiatives that went nowhere.[37] In particular, the African American community was continuously marginalized, segregated from white residents, and placed into circumstances that perpetuated the trend of poverty, unemployment, and high crime. By the time the 2008 financial crisis hit the rest of the country, Flint was already barely staying above water, and the repeated broken promises and declining conditions created an environment toxic to a trusting relationship between Flint and its political and administrative leaders.

The Newest Chapter

The City of Flint found itself in such a dire financial situation that from 2002 to 2006, and again in 2011, Governor Snyder appointed an emergency financial manager (renamed an emergency manager under new legislation in 2012), using the controversial state law allowing him to appoint a single manager with sweeping unilateral powers over municipal decisions without any requirement for input or approval of the democratically elected city officials.[38] In 2013, the city decided to join a new regional system for drinking water rather than continue to buy its water from Detroit. Rather than continue paying for water from Detroit while the regional system was built, city officials decided to switch the city to water from the Flint River. Emergency manager Darnell Earley oversaw the switch. As has been well-documented, this decision proved catastrophic. The city did not control for the corrosive quality of the water coming from the Flint River, which allowed the water to leach lead from the network of lead pipes crisscrossing the city.[39]

While the elevated levels of lead have received the most attention due to the disastrous effects lead has on the health of children, lead was not the first problem to emerge. Immediately after switching to the Flint River water, residents began complaining about the water from their taps coming out murky and brown, often with a foul odor. Over the first few months, several boil orders were announced to Flint residents because of bacteria such as E. coli that had been found in samples across the city. Residents noticed rashes, stomach problems, hair loss, and other physical problems presenting in adults and children across the area. Many citizens attended the public forums held by the emergency manager to voice their concerns and call on officials to do something to fix the situation. State and city officials repeatedly told them that the water met federal standards, and their concerns were dismissed.[40]

While much of the literature focuses on service delivery and the quality of these services affecting trust between the public and the government, in the case of Flint, residents had already become accustomed to crumbling infrastructure, high fees, and a lack of resources. Some stayed out of a love for their community; many more stayed because they were unable to sell their houses and could not afford to move elsewhere. In the case of Flint, the water from the tap was ruining their physical health, but it was the treatment by officials at the city, state, and national levels that poisoned their relationship with government. One resident at the time, LeeAnne Walters, whose concerns continually fell on deaf ears, decided to research water testing on her own. Based on her own understanding of the process, she discovered that what the emergency manager and officials from the Michigan Department of Environmental Quality (MDEQ) were telling her could not be accurate. As many media outlets and the Flint Water Advisory Task Force (FWATF) have shown, the MDEQ testing was problematic from the beginning, with a flawed sample protocol which did not include the most at-risk homes in Flint, followed by changes to the sample selection protocol partway through the process, and inaccurate directions given to residents collecting water from the tap in their homes. Walters had water from her home tested by the city, and the levels of lead were alarmingly high. After receiving these results and contacting city officials, Walters was first told the lead must be coming from the pipes on her property—which would remove any responsibility on the part of the city—but this proved impossible because the pipes in her home had been replaced with plastic pipes several years earlier. "Walters says that when she brought her concerns to city officials, they told her that they were following the law, and if she had a problem, she could take it up with the [Environmental Protection Agency (EPA)]. So, she did."[41]

Walters contacted EPA employee Miguel Del Toral, as well as Marc Edwards, a civil engineer and expert on corrosion control at Virginia Tech. This was the turning point—city and state officials had repeatedly ignored citizen concerns, but with the attention garnered by Edwards and Del Toral, as well as the work of local physician Mona Hanna-Attisha to analyze the lead levels of children throughout Flint, the story began to receive national attention. Much to the anger and frustration of residents, after endless months of their own claims that something was wrong being ignored, it was outsiders who brought the situation to a crisis point. Governor Snyder declared a state of emergency, investigations into the actions of government officials began, and the fallout continues as employees at all levels concerned with Flint have resigned. As of June 2017, fifteen current and former state and local employees have been charged with misleading federal regulatory officials, manipulating water sampling, tampering with reports, and involuntary manslaughter.[42]

The results of testing by Edwards and his colleagues provided vindication to the residents of Flint. A graduate student working with Edwards contacted residents whose samples had tested high for lead, and the reactions of those he contacted speak volumes: "One woman said to us, 'You mean that's the results for my tap? That's empowering.'"[43] After over a year of being told by public officials that her own experience, the tangible evidence that she saw every day, was within federal guidelines and should not be a concern, she finally had validation.

Even as criminal charges continue to be filed, and the national spotlight continues to shine on Flint, residents express their frustrations. Some claim they will not feel that justice has been done until the emergency manager, Earley, is held responsible for his decision to use the Flint River; others believe that Governor Snyder should face charges, despite his continued statements that he was not aware of the situation as it was.[44] Part of the trust relationship between citizens and their government comes from the ability of citizens to hold public officials accountable, the option for them to "throw the rascals out" should their decisions and actions not demonstrate that they are upholding their end of the political bargain.[45] The use of an emergency manager, a controversial measure in Michigan, placed the residents of Flint in a position of disenfranchisement, disempowered from actively participating in the workings of their government. The emergency manager law itself was passed by the Michigan legislature with a provision that the public could not revoke the measure, and so from the state level down to the residents of Flint, political power and the ability to hold their government accountable was removed from the beginning.[46]

When citizens cannot hold their government accountable, when their voices are removed from the process and their concerns ignored, and when their experiences conflict with the information obtained from the state itself, what little trust may have existed is eroded even further. Flint's political history of disenfranchisement and broken promises created a distrustful environment, and the actions of officials in the most recent water crisis have continued the iterative negative process by which trust is lost. The use of an emergency manager removed power from the citizens of Flint, and spurred a manmade crisis setting Flint apart from other cities struggling with economic insecurity and declining infrastructure. Government officials responded to the personal experiences of Flint residents by dismissing them and obscuring vital information. Blame continues to be shuffled between several agencies and all levels of government, making it is no surprise that the media narrative continues to focus on how public trust has been demolished, and how citizens are not sure if they can ever trust government officials again.

As government officials attempt to address the situation, this level of distrust impedes even those whose actions finally forced the government to admit that a problem existed. Laura Sullivan, a water expert at Kettering University in Flint, finds that even as a local source of information, she faces wary citizens as she advises them on water safety, because she is now working with officials from Snyder's administration.[47] Officials have instructed some areas of the city that the water, which is once again coming from Detroit, is safe to drink; even so, residents are buying bottled water due to their unwillingness to trust the information they are receiving. Those who cannot afford bottled water visit friends or family members in the suburbs to use their water, while still paying some of the highest prices in the country for the water coming into their homes. City officials asked state and federal agencies for funding to replace the lead pipes in the city.[48] An ensuing legal settlement required the state to comply, and pipe replacement is almost complete as of 2020.

The literature on trust within public administration has focused on the trust relationship between the public and bureaucrats, with the assumption that these public officials are doing the best that they can in a constrained environment, and should focus on ways in which administrators can be open and transparent with the public to increase trust.[49] What Flint has shown, however, is that we need to begin to consider the issue of trust in situations where the foundations of trust are already failing, as well as situations where public managers actively fail the public. In cities across the country, we see communities like Flint's continuing to be marginalized, dismissed, and sometimes actively harmed due to the inaction or lack of caring on the part of those who are in charge of their health and safety. When a state of emergency occurs because of the callousness of those at the top, researchers need to start asking how such a system can ever be considered legitimate and trustworthy again.

Conclusion

In 1945, a General Motors (GM) historian for the Buick division of the company published a book on the relationship the company shared with its hometown of Flint, Michigan, entitled *The City of Flint Grows Up*. The glowing tome served as a tribute to the mutually beneficial relationship between the company and the town that had led to the industrial supremacy of GM and the prosperity of Flint, the shining example of the American Dream in action. "Buick is Flint and Flint is Buick" was a phrase adopted by the historian Carl Crow, who concluded that "America is a thousand Flints," as he and the rest of the nation celebrated the booming economy in the post-war land of progress, prosperity and opportunity.[50]

Now, comfortably into the 21st century, Crow's conclusions seem oddly prophetic. After the economic turmoil of 2008 caused the great auto manufacturers in the country to claim bankruptcy, it appears that Flint is in fact Buick. Tied for nearly a decade to the success of GM, the once-booming town of Flint has fallen further and further into decline and now faces an environmental health crisis of epic proportions. The switch from the Detroit water system to the Flint River as the source for municipal water has resulted in numerous health scares, and alarmingly high levels of lead in the blood of Flint's children; but in this way, Flint is not alone. Across the country, urban centers, often in similar dire economic straits, have found themselves struggling to provide the most basic of services such as clean water to the increasingly impoverished citizenry that remain. Due to years of leaded gasoline and lead paint, children in urban areas routinely exhibit high levels of lead in their blood from exposure to contaminated soil and housing, a problem that is beyond the capacity of local governments to address (Nelson 2016). While each struggling city has a unique story of decline, each can be seen as a microcosm of the increasingly distrustful public that continues to look upon government with skepticism and disdain. With each report of high levels of lead, each leaked e-mail showing a lack of responsiveness, each use of state authority to remove the ability for citizens to self-govern, Flint and every other city like it moves towards the precipice of a crisis of trust.

Notes

1. Robbins, Denise. "Analysis: How Michigan and national reporters cover the Flint water crisis," *Media Matters for America*, February 2, 2016.

2. Ibid.

3. Davis, Matthew M., Chris Kolb, Lawrence Reynolds, Eric Rothstein and Ken Sikkema. "Flint Water Advisory Task Force Final Report." 2016. Office of Governor Rick Snyder, State of Michigan.

4. Hetherington, Marc J. 1998. "The political relevance of political trust." *American Political Science Review*, 92 (4): 791-808.

5. Ibid.; Pew Research Center, November 2015. "Beyond distrust: How Americans view their government." Pew Research Center.

6. Hetherington, 1998; Levi, Margaret and Laura Stoker. 2000. "Political trust and trustworthiness." *Annual Review of Political Science*, 3: 475-507.

7. Easton, David. 1965. *A systems analysis of political life*. New York: Wiley.

8. Berman, Evan M. 1997. "Dealing with Cynical Citizens." *Public Administration Review*, 57 (2): 105-112; Cook, Timothy and Paul Gronke. 2005. "Skeptical American: Revisiting the meanings of trust in government and confidence in institutions." *Journal of Politics*, 67 (3): 784-803.

9. Belanger, Eric and Richard Nadeau. 2005. "Political trust and the vote in multiparty elections: The Canadian case." *European Journal of Political Research*, 44: 121-146; Citrin, Jack. 1996. "Who's the Boss? Direct Democracy and Popular Control of Government." In *Broken Contract: Changing Relationships Between Americans and Their Government*, ed. Stephen C. Craig. Boulder, CO: Westview; Citrin, Jack, and Donald Philip Green. 1986. "Presidential Leadership and the Resurgence of Trust in Government." *British Journal of Political Science* 16 (October): 431-53; Hetherington, 1998; Hetherington. 1999. "The effect of political trust on the presidential vote, 1968-1996." *American Political Science Review* 93 (2): 311-326; Miller, Arthur H. and Stephen A. Borrelli. 1991. "Confidence in government during the 1980s." *American Politics Research* 19 (2): 147-173.

10. Craig, Stephen C. 1996. "Change and the American Electorate." In *Broken Contract: Changing Relationships Between Americans and Their Government*, ed. Stephen C. Craig. Boulder, CO: Westview; Miller, Arthur H. 1974. "Political Issues and Trust in Government, 1964-70." *American Political Science Review* 68 (September): 951-72.

11. Levi and Stoker, 2000.

12. Hetherington, 1998.

13. Hetherington, Marc J. and Thomas J. Rudolph. 2008. "Priming, performance, and the dynamics of political trust." *Journal of Politics* 70 (2): 498-512.

14. Hetherington, 1998.

15. Levi, Margaret. 1988. *Of rule and revenue*. Berkeley: University of California Press; Levi, Margaret. 1997. *Consent, dissent and patriotism*. New York: Cambridge University Press..; Levi and Stokes, 2000; Marien, Sofie, and Marc

Hooghe. 2011. "Does political trust matter? An empirical investigation into the relation between political trust and support for law compliance." *European Journal of Political Research* 50: 267-291; Tyler, Tom R. 1990. *Why people obey the law.* New Haven, CT: Yale University Press.

16. Rahn, Wendy M. and Thomas J. Rudolph. 2005. "A tale of political trust in American cities." *Public Opinion Quarterly* 69 (4): 530-560.

17. Cooper, Christopher A., H. Gibbs Knotts and Kathleen M. Brennan. 2008. "The Importance of Trust in Government for Public Administration: The Case of Zoning." *Public Administration Review* 68 (3): 459-468; Rahn and Rudolph, 2005.

18. Rahn and Rudolph, 2005.

19. Berman, 1997.

20. Satterfield, Terre, C.K. Mertz, and Paul Slovic. 2004. "Discrimination, vulnerability, and justice in the face of risk." *Risk Analysis* 24 (1): 115-129.

21. Stivers, Camilla. 2007. "'So poor and so black': Hurricane Katrina, public administration, and the issue of race." *Public Administration Review* 67 (Supplements 1): 48-56.

22. Ibid.

23. Maynard-Moody, Steven, and Michael Musheno. 2003. *Cops, Teachers, Counselors: Stories from the Front Lines of Public Service.* Ann Arbor: University of Michigan Press.

24. Scammell, Madeleine Kangsen, Laura Senier, Jennifer Darrah-Okike, Phil Brown, and Susan Santos. 2009. "Tangible evidence, trust and power: Public perceptions of community environmental health studies." *Social Science and Medicine* 68: 140-153.

25. Davis, et al., 2016.

26. Office of the Governor. "Gov. Rick Snyder announces Flint Water Task," *State of Michigan Office of the Governor.* October 21, 2015.

27. Barry-Jester, Anna Maria. "What went wrong in Flint," *FiveThirtyEight*, January 26, 2016; Gleick, Peter and Marc Edwards. "One step to help restore trust in Flint," *Detroit Free Press*, March 6, 2016; Groden, Claire. "How Michigan's bureaucrats created the Flint water crisis," *Fortune*, n.d.; Nelson, Libby. "The Flint water crisis, explained," *Vox*, February 15, 2016; Robbins, Denise. "Analysis: How Michigan and national reporters cover the Flint water crisis," *Media Matters for America*, February 2, 2016; Sell, Sarah. "Emotional testimony about Flint water crisis," *ABC WZZM 13*, March 29, 2016; Shapiro, Ari. "Flint res-

idents' broken faith: "The people we trusted failed us,'" NPR, February 10, 2016; Simon, Mallory and Sara Sidner. "Flint water crisis: Families bear scars from 'manmade disaster,'" CNN, March 5, 2016.

28. Highsmith, Andrew R. 2015. *Demolition means progress: Flint, Michigan and the fate of the American metropolis.* Chicago, IL: University of Chicago Press.

29. Davis, et al., 2016.

30. Scammell, et al., 2009.

31. Stivers, 2007.

32. Highsmith, 2015.

33. Ibid.

34. Ibid.

35. Ibid.

36. Highsmith, 2016.

37. Highsmith, 2015.

38. Michigan Radio Newsroom. "7 things to know about Michigan's emergency manager law," *Michigan Radio*, December 6, 2011.

39. Barry-Jester, 2016; Nelson, 2016.

40. Barry-Jester, 2016.

41. Ibid.

42. Atkinson, Scott and Monica Davey. "5 charged with involuntary manslaughter in Flint water crisis," New York Times, June 14, 2017; McLaughlin, Eliott C. and Catherine E. Scholchet. "Charges against 3 in Flint water crisis 'only the beginning,'" CNN, April 20, 2016.

43. Barry-Jester, 2016.

44. McLaughlin and Scholchet, 2016.

45. Belanger and Nadeau, 2005; Hetherington, 1999.

46. Michigan Radio Newsroom, 2011.

47. Shapiro, 2016.

48. Fantz, Ashley and Kristina Sgueglia. "Flint mayor says $55 million needed to replace lead pipes." CNN, February 9, 2016; Simon and Sidner, 2016.

49. Berg, Anne Marie. 2005. "Creating Trust? A critical perspective on trust-enhancing efforts in public services." *Public Performance and Management Review* 28 (4): 465-486.

50. Highsmith, 2015.

CHAPTER 3

AUTHORIZATION OF EMERGENCY FINANCIAL MANAGERS DURING FLINT

Jeremy N. Phillips

Introduction

As the events leading up to the Flint Water Crisis unfolded, the citizens of Flint, Michigan, lacked a democratically-elected entity to represent their interests related to fiscal matters, and instead were subject to the fiats of a state-approved Emergency Manager (EM). EMs were known as Emergency Financial Managers (EFMs) prior to enactment of Public Act 436, discussed in more detail below. Michigan stands apart from most states in the U.S. in that EMs act in place of elected leaders. As testament to this point, on August 21, 2012, Edward Kurtz, the appointed Emergency Manager of Flint, Michigan, at the time, signed Order No. 3 and outlined the authority of the EM, which reads:

> ... the [EM has the] authority and responsibilities of the Mayor and City Councils concerning the adoption, amendment, and enforcement of ordinances and resolutions affecting the financial condition of the City of Flint; and ... has the authority to approve or disapprove all outstanding financial obligations ... and ... has the authority to amend, revise, approve, or disapprove the budget ... and limit the total amount appropriated or expended during the balance of the financial emergency ....

For four years the City of Flint's financial decision making rested in the hands of state appointed EMs. Not only are these individuals credited for setting the water crisis into motion, but their decisions created additional economic, physical, and emotional difficulties for the residents of Flint.

Michigan is not the only state with statutes to handle fiscal emergencies of local governments. They are, however, at the forefront a growing trend to give appointed administrators unprecedented power to govern fiscal matters. Using Flint as a case study, the authors present evidence that Michigan's fiscal emergencies statutes can exacerbate troubles in a community because they 1) eliminate democratic decision making, 2) lack transparency, 3) task EMs to correct financial situations they often have limited ability to affect, and 4) incentivize short-term solutions over the long-term needs of a community. Given these characteristics, states that pursue EM policies similar to Michigan's risk public health and safety catastrophes similar to those experienced by Flint's residents.

The chapter is organized as follows. The authors begin by laying out a working definition of what constitutes a fiscal crisis. From there, they review various approaches of states to deal with local governmental fiscal crises. An overview of Michigan's EM law is provided, with particular attention to the appropriateness of the law in helping Flint overcome its fiscal crisis. It is in this section that the authors make the case that Michigan's EM law was inadequate to help Flint make a long-term recovery, assaulted democratic ideals, and undermined public safety. The authors conclude the chapter by offering suggestions for alternative approaches for state lawmakers to consider.

Overview of Municipal and State Responses to Fiscal Crises

State lawmakers nationwide have various options at their disposal to respond to fiscal challenges. To gain a better understanding of the severity of Michigan's EM provision, it is appropriate to review available actions that other states have used to deal with fiscal crisis. The sections below review common approaches, starting with constructing a working definition of fiscal crisis.

Defining a Fiscal Crisis. Oftentimes fiscal stress and fiscal crisis are used interchangeably; however, in order to clarify the State's role in the process, it is important to highlight the distinction. Fiscal stress is common for governments. When the economic environment is altered in some way, such as a recession or change in tax base, governments often experience a budgetary strain. This is especially true for smaller governments that lack revenue diversification. The key distinction between fiscal stress and a crisis is that fiscal stress is temporary, and may be remedied through changes in the tax structure, expenditure cuts, or utilization of reserve funds or credit lines.

Municipalities pass the threshold of fiscal crisis when budgetary flexibility disappears. A government faces a crisis when "no combination of acceptable expenditure cuts, revenue increases, and borrowing exists."[1] Moreover, fiscal crises are pervasive and remedies often lie beyond the abilities of the local government to correct on their own. To be sure, there is overlap between stress and a crisis, and oftentimes fiscal stress is the precursor to a crisis, but the distinction is important because a fiscal crisis often requires assistance and guidance from the state.

Causes of a Fiscal Crisis. The strategies states adopt to deal with fiscal crises are largely influenced by the cause. An analysis of the state's response to local government fiscal crises found the most common cause of a crisis was attributable to local economic conditions. Although downturns in the economy are temporary, they can have profound effects on smaller governments. Smaller municipalities are less likely to draw from a diversified tax base and instead rely primarily on a single industry or employer, which can have devastating fiscal implications for the locality if altered.[2] In a similar vein, changes in population and the demographic composition of a population can strain the budget.[3] For example, a municipality's tax base will be impacted if residents move outside of a jurisdiction, property values decline, or annual income of the residents decline. Reductions in intergovernmental revenues and unfunded mandates have also left many local governments with sizable budget gaps. It should also be noted that fiscal mismanagement and political disagreements about how to deal with budget shortfalls exacerbate fiscal problems.

Responding to a Fiscal Crisis. A 2003 study identified four broad categories for dealing with local government fiscal crisis, which include predicting, averting, mitigating, and preventing the recurrence of a fiscal crisis.[4] These strategies can range from heavy-handed approaches, such as state takeovers, to softer measures such as serving as a technical advisor.[5]

Taking a proactive response to a fiscal crisis, states use a variety of sources to predict and, theoretically, prevent an impending fiscal crisis.[6] State officials use audit reports, local government reports and publications, as well as data generated by special monitoring systems to help identify an issue before a government enters into a fiscal crisis. Closely related to prediction, averting a fiscal crisis involves state officials taking action to help the local government avoid the catastrophe. Several states have established debt, expenditure, and investment limits, as well as formal rules related to auditing, reporting, and monitoring meant to establish avoid a fiscal crisis. These laws prevent local governments from engaging in behavior that can cause a fiscal crisis and supply information for the state to monitor financial conditions.

If state officials determine a crisis is imminent, they intervene with technical assistance or recommendations to the municipality.[7] More assertive measures include diverting funds to pay debt obligations, mandating local governments lay off employees, cutting expenditures, or raising taxes (Honadle, 2003).[8]

Actions related to mitigating a fiscal crisis tend to be much more "hands on" and involve direct actions to reestablish financial solvency. Honadle (2003) finds that mitigation efforts are more common than prevention, a trend she attributes to a lack of formal prevention rules.[9] Additionally, since a fiscal crisis has implication beyond the government experiencing the crisis, state officials have a motivation to take corrective action. States generally provide technical, managerial, and financial assistance when trying to mitigate the crisis. Other actions include state approval of future budgets, instituting control boards, placing the local government in receivership, drafting recovery plans, and relaxing laws related to debt and revenue limitations.[10]

After the fiscal crisis has past, some states continue to monitor the fiscal matters of the municipality to avoid the reoccurrence of a fiscal crisis. Specific actions taken during the monitoring phase are similar to what is described above, the difference being the municipality has moved beyond the crisis.[11]

How Does Michigan Handle Fiscal Emergencies?

Laying out Michigan's Emergency Manager law is difficult because the state enacted different versions of the law during Flint's receivership. This section details the EM laws that initially governed Flint. In the concluding section of this chapter, the latest version of the law is reviewed.

Michigan law pertaining to local government fiscal crisis began in 1988 with Public Act 101, which was designed to deal with a financial emergency in Hamtramck, MI. Public Act 101 was replaced and expanded with Public Act 72 of 1990. The justification of the expansion reads as follows:

> ... the public health and welfare of the citizens of this state would be adversely affected by the insolvency of units of local government ... and that the survival of units of local government is vitally necessary to the interest of the people of this state to provide necessary governmental services. The legislature further determines that it is vitally

38

necessary to protect the credit of the state and its political subdivision and that it is a valid public purpose for the state to take action and to assist a unit of local government in a fiscal emergency situation to remedy this emergency situation by required prudent fiscal management ...

Public Act 72 lays out 14 different "triggers" to alert state officials to a potential emergency financial situation. To summarize, the state treasurer can conduct a preliminary analysis to determine if a local unit is suffering a fiscal crisis if 1) the state treasurer receives a request for review from members of a governing body, 2) if the local government fails to meet obligations to creditors, pensioners, or employees, or 3) if the local government fails to comply with other state laws related to fiscal matters.

Many of these triggers signify a proactive approach. While the triggers laid out in the statute do not fall into the category of "predictive," the law is written in a manner that allows the state to intervene early and take actions to avert a crisis. A review can be requested if interested parties have concerns and/or the local government does not uphold their financial obligations. Additionally, the state has a variety of fiscal compliance mechanisms that, if not met, raise concerns about the fiscal health the local government.

If the state treasurer finds evidence of a serious financial problem, the governor appoints a financial team to conduct a more detailed review. In addition to reviewing necessary documents, the review team has the authority to sign a consent agreement with the chief administrative officer that specifies necessary actions for recovery. This agreement, which must be approved by local officials, includes provisions for technical assistance, strategies to balance the local government's budget, schedules for debt payment, and/or additional reporting requirements.

Actions of the fiscal review team can be seen as both averting and mitigating a financial crisis. The law is written in a way that encourages proactive behavior of the state treasurer when potential for a financial crisis arises. And, as will be evident below, the consent agreement can be a powerful tool to avoid receivership.

If the review team is not able draw up a satisfactory plan, or the local government does not follow through with the agreement, then the governor may assign a local emergency financial assistance loan board to oversee the municipality's fiscal affairs. This board then appoints an EFM. Under Public Act 72, the EFM has a broad range of authority to oversee local government operations, including the power to act in place of all government officials and elected leaders; to amend, approve, or disapprove the budget; to layoff and/or adjust pay for employees and elected officials; to establish a plan for repaying obligations; to cancel government services; to enter into contracts for services with private organizations or other governments; to sell government assets; to renegotiate labor contracts, and act as the local government's designee in labor negotiations; and to apply for loans on behalf of the local governments. It should also be noted while that while there are no residency requirements for the EFM, the local government must pay the EFM's salary. Also of special note, the EFM cannot impose a tax increase.

Passed in 2011, Public Act 4 expanded the EFM law established with PA 72. The most notable changes were to the "triggers," making it easier for the State Treasurer to initiate a review. Additionally, the EFM was given the authority to adjust and terminate collective bargaining agreements and make adjustments to pensions under certain circumstances.

Public Act 4 was quickly rejected by Michigan voters by referendum.[12] Lawmakers responded with Public Act 436, which now governs local financial emergencies in Michigan. This new law addresses many of the criticisms levied at PA 72 and PA 4, namely, that the previous statutes limited the options of local governments experiencing a financial crisis and that those options placed a disproportionate burden on citizens and employees. In response, the new law gave local governing bodies more say in the process. In the concluding sections of this chapter, the authors highlight the positives of the new law.

Analysis of Flint

For any policy to have sufficient impact, it must be designed in a way that fits the reality of the situation. Undoubtedly, EMs are appropriate when municipalities face severe fiscal stress and clear paths to the solution are apparent. Yet when the municipality has taken appropriate steps to deal with their fiscal situation, but structural deficits exist, there is little an EM can do to help. In fact, in such a situation an EM can do more harm than good.

As detailed in the coming paragraphs, leading up to the state takeover in 2011, Flint experienced major deficits due to structural and cyclical factors.

In addition to a major national recession, over the last decade Flint underwent a significant erosion of their tax base, coupled with a major reduction in city's labor market, and rising personnel and pension costs. Moreover, Michigan statutes eliminated most options for the city to proactively increase revenues, while simultaneously reducing financial support due to the state's own budgetary shortfall.

Demographic and Financial Overview of Flint

Population Changes. Information compiled over the past four decades reflects that Flint has experienced serious population declines, dropping from a population of 197,000 in 1960 to approximately 102,000 in 2010.[14] This population loss seems to have quickened in the recent past with a decline of 18% between 2000 and 2010. Moreover, the flight from Flint breaks along racial and class lines. In 1960, the population of Flint was roughly 162,000 white and 35,000 black. In 2010, the population was 38,000 white and 58,000 black. Flint has also experienced significant changes in composition of wealth living in the jurisdiction. In 1970, about 12% of Flint's population lived below the poverty below the federal poverty level. By 2009, roughly 35% of city residents had household incomes below the poverty line.

Employment Changes. There have also been significant changes in employment within Flint. Again, using data compiled in 2001, the ten largest employers in Flint offered 51,546 jobs.[15] Ten years later, the number of jobs offered by these same employers had declined to 38,022. With few new employers coming into Flint, the overall number of jobs in the city dropped from 90,412 in 2001 to 49,500 by 2010.

The job loss naturally contributed to the unemployment rates in the city. Flint consistently had an unemployment rate 1-2% higher than the state average between 2000-2010. In the two years leading up to the state takeover of Flint, the average annual unemployment rate in Flint 14.9% in 2009 and 14.0% in 2010.

Tax Revenues. The City of Flint's Comprehensive Annual Financial Report (CAFR) reveals that the three primary tax revenue sources, totaling 72% of Flint's general fund, are state shared revenue (31%), income tax (24%), property tax (17%). Similar to the city's demographic trends, Flint's tax bases have eroded in the recent past. State shared revenues declined by 13%, dropping from $20,040,661 to $17,446,231, between 2006 and 2010.

41

Unfortunately, in Flint, state shared revenue is both constitutionally and statutorily defined, which limits the city's ability to mitigate the situation. The constitutional provision parses out payments based on population, and as noted above, Flint has experienced a substantial decrease in population. The statutory provision distributes payments based on a formula; however, the State of Michigan has not fully funded the statutory portion in over a decade.[16] The fact that state lawmakers did not meet their statutory obligations is not surprising because payments to other governments entities are typically one of the first things cut in times of fiscal stress.

Income tax revenue is the second largest source of revenue for Flint, and this declined by 31% from $19,660,536 in 2006 to $13,551,127 in 2010. Increases in unemployment and the flight of employers from Flint are largely responsible for the $6 million dollars loss in income tax revenue. However, according to the Flint City Treasurer, raising the income tax by .05% for city residents and .25% for non-residents would generate approximately $6.6 million, making up the revenue lost to population changes;[17] raising income tax is possible only with the consent of the state legislature.

As with the other major revenue sources, property tax revenue experienced significant losses between 2006 and 2010, declining by 24% from $12,540,496 in 2006 to $9,474,168 in 2010. Much of this drop can be attributed to the exodus from Flint, which has dramatically increased the number of vacant homes. Some estimate 10,849 homes, nearly 61% of Flint's entire housing stock in 2010, stand vacant.[18] Despite the dire circumstances, Flint had limited options because, like the income tax provision, the State of Michigan restricts the taxable value and multiplier used to calculate property tax.

Expenditures. Reviewing Flint's expenditures reveals that the city has made substantial efforts to reduce its expenses. Like most governments, personnel costs make up the majority of Flint's expenditures. Flint reduced the number of employees from 1,526 in 2001 to 767 in 2010. To highlight the severity of the cuts, in 2001 the city employed 336 sworn officers. This number was reduced to 122 by 2010.[19] Despite these dramatic cuts in personnel, costs related to rising healthcare and pension obligations limited the impact of personnel cuts.[20]

A common suggestion for governments experiencing fiscal issues is to outsource services to the private sector. However, a study on Michigan municipalities noted that Flint/s city government had very few services which could be outsourced.[21]

The Appropriateness of Michigan's EM Law

The application of Michigan's EM law in Flint should serve as a warning to other state leaders as they grapple with how to deal with local-level fiscal crises. The structure of Michigan's EFM under Public Act 72, and especially Public Act 4, was not only inappropriate to deal with the financial crisis experienced in Flint, but arguably put the health and welfare of citizens at risk by incentivized myopic decision making and willful disregard for democratic ideals and local autonomy.

The Response Did Not Fit the Situation. An EM is advantageous in that the person can help lawmakers decide who should bear the impact of tax increases and/or cuts to services in order to alleviate the fiscal crisis.[22] This, of course, assumes that tough choices can actually fix the fiscal crisis, and after examining the structural issues facing Flint, one has to wonder how an EM could have helped. In the year leading up to the state takeover, Flint had a general fund deficit of $14.6 million and a total long term debt of $155.8 million, not including an underfunded pension obligation.[23] While the EM can request support from the state, he/she cannot make state lawmakers restore cuts to state revenue sharing. Likewise, the EM cannot impose tax increases without special approval from the state. Even if the EM could increase taxes, they faced with a declining population, declining property values, and a significant population that did not have the financial means to bear an increase in tax burden.

Cutting expenditures to alleviate the financial crisis was not an option, either. Recall, the city cut its personnel by more than half prior to entering receivership. The city still has an obligation to provide essential services to its citizens. Flint still had the same grounds to keep, sewer lines to maintain, and roads to patrol. And, as will be discussed below, further attempts to reduce expenditures made by the EFM had significant consequences for the residents of Flint.

In summary, there was little the EM could do in Flint to help solve the problem. To be sure, the EM could, and did, find ways to save additional money; however, Flint faced major structural deficits which were beyond the capabilities of the EM to remedy. As we argue below, receivership under Michigan law promotes a short-term solutions at the expense of public health and safety, and strips the local government of democracy and local autonomy principals.

Incentivizes Short Term Decisions. The governor selects an individual to solve the financial crisis as quickly as possible. To do this, the EM can act unilaterally and in lieu of all elected officials. Taken together, this sets the stage for decisions that are not in the long-term interest of the community. For example, in 2009, Pontiac's EM auctioned the Silverdome, the former Detroit Lions' stadium, for $583,000 to bring in extra cash. Yet a year before the city had received (but rejected) a $20 million bid for the same stadium (*New Orleans Business Review*, 2009).[24]

Moreover, during the Flint water crisis, Congressional testimony from the then-presiding EM suggests the decision to switch water sources was motivated, in part, by potential cost savings. One wonders if locally-elected officials would have made the same decision. The take-away point is this—in an effort to carry out their duties, the structure of Michigan's EM rewards short-term financial decisions rather than the pursuit of long-term solutions in the best interest of the community.

Risk to Public Safety and Quality of Life. Building off of the arguments above, when the long-term needs of the community take a back seat, public safety and quality of life are put at risk. Consider the aforementioned cut in sworn officers—by 2010, "Flint employ[ed] one officer for about every 830 people. Comparatively, New York City (which didn't even make the top 25 most dangerous cities) covers about 235 people per cop."[25]

As one would expect, these cuts were made in the name of correcting the fiscal crisis with little regard to the dangerous repercussions. As a result, Flint has held a spot in the top 5 most violent cities for several years in a row and is recognized as one of the most dangerous cities in the U.S. for women.[26]

Cuts to other areas of Flint's government, such as Parks and Recreation and Public Works, were just as dramatic, and arguably decreased the quality of life for Flint residents. For example, in 2009 Flint employed 11 administrators and 13 groundskeepers in the Parks and Recreation Department. By 2014, these divisions were gutted to one employee each. Similarly, street maintenance dropped from 36 employees in 2009 to 16 in 2014.[27]

Lack of Democratic Ideals, Local Autonomy, and Transparency. Under Michigan Law, the EM serves in place of locally-elected officials. We have demonstrated that this provision gives the EM unilateral authority, removing local residents' voices in the decisions that impact their community. Moreover, these EM operate in relative secrecy, exempt from the state's open meeting laws and not subject to the same level of transparency through open records.[28]

To demonstrate the assault on democratic ideals, local autonomy, and transparency, one only needs to look to the orders issued by Michael Brown, Flint's first EM. In his first days on the job, Mr. Brown eliminated the salaries and benefits of the mayor and city council, and terminated the appointments of numerous administrators. Although a portion of the mayor and council members' compensation was later restored, Mr. Brown's executive orders sent a clear message that both the mayor and council members serve at the pleasure of the EM.[29] As noted by Mlive, "under the state law governing state takeovers, elected office holder are prohibited from exercising authority without permission of the emergency manager."[30]

Mr. Brown also canceled city council meetings until further notice.[31] While he did restore the public meetings later, Mr. Brown still constrained the democratic process by reducing the number of from twice- to once-a-month. Executive Order No. 12 provides further insight into Mr. Brown's opinion of democracy in Flint. In order to address the City Council, members of the public must submit a written question prior to the start of the meeting. In fact, residents are restricted to one comment per period, which may not exceed five minutes.

A Better Path for Flint

It can be argued that city and state officials may have discounted the advantages provided by Chapter 9 of the U.S. Bankruptcy Code. Recent municipal bankruptcy rulings in Stockton, CA and Detroit, MI demonstrated that the Code ensures the continuation of essential services and may represent a more democratic path than the EM. After the citizens of Michigan voted against Public Act 4, lawmakers replaced it with Public Act 436, which gave municipalities more flexibility in dealing with a financial crisis. One option now available for municipalities is Chapter 9.

As the only form of bankruptcy permitted under the U.S. Bankruptcy Code for municipalities, Chapter 9 offers some unique provisions. For example, municipalities have the exclusive right to propose debt restructuring plans to the bankruptcy court during the automatic stay period.[32] Protection under Chapter 9 also ensures that control over the municipality remains in local hands. In other words, the bankruptcy code prevents the assignation of a trustee to oversee the municipality and prohibits the bankruptcy court from instructing local authorities to take any action.[33] Related to this point, Chapter 9 proscribes creditors from taking municipal property as payment, as well as bans municipalities from liquidating their assets.[34]

Perhaps most importantly, Chapter 9 contains a provision that ensures continuation of the municipality's infrastructure, as well as the safety of its residents.[35] The rulings in Detroit and Stockton have strengthened this feature by declaring that public health and safety must be considered during the debt negotiation process. Moreover, these rulings suggest the taxpayers of Flint may be considered a "party of interest" and thus a special form of creditors. This opens up the debt readjustment process to the citizens of the municipality, ultimately giving them a voice in the bankruptcy process.

However, bankruptcy has many costs that city officials must consider. First, the city assumes increased borrowing costs due to a decrease in credit ratings, as credit markets will undoubtedly downgrade, if not suspend, the municipality's credit.[36] Municipalities will also incur significant legal fees—potentially in the seven figures—as they will require counsel not only to trigger the proceedings, but also during the creditors' potential challenges during the filing and the automatic stay, as well as the debt negotiations.[37] Further, an insolvent municipality may be a social stigma, negatively impacting the psychological health of the residents, as well as the business climate.[38] Lastly, the bankruptcy may not address root causes of the fiscal crisis. If the municipality does not address the underlying issue, the problems will "continue to haunt" the municipality after it emerges from bankruptcy.[39]

In Michigan, there are additional costs to the process, as state law requires that the municipality to enter receivership prior to filing. The EM must then petition the Local Emergency Financial Assistance Loan Board, which then forwards it to the governor for final approval.

Finally, a few questions remain regarding the strength of the Detroit's rulings, as well as Flint's eligibility for Chapter 9. Traditionally, a municipality had to meet five conditions to qualify for Chapter 9, one of which is insolvency. However, Detroit and Stockton solidified the concepts of "service delivery insolvency," or the inability to provide essential services to residents.[40] At this point in the Flint water crisis, it is no secret that Flint failed in its compact to provide services to its residents.

In sum, Chapter 9 ensures the continuation of essential municipal services and, if the recent rulings stand, may prove to be a more transparent and democratic process for taxpayers. It is hoped that policymakers fully consider the costs and benefits of the process when a municipality faces a similar situation as Flint.

Conclusion

As more states formalize policies to deal with local government financial emergencies, Flint should serve as an example for the need to design policies that address the root cause of the emergency while also preserving the integrity of the local community. Financial emergencies are brought on by a variety of factors, and EM laws should be designed to allow officials to specifically address these factors. In passing Public Act 436, Michigan took a step to abide by these suggestions. Local communities now have several paths to address and overcome their specific financial emergencies. Additionally, Public Act 436 allows local communities to have a voice in the process.

Notes

1.   Hirsch, Werner Zvi, and Anthony M Rufolo. 1990. *Public finance and expenditure in a federal system*: Harcourt College Pub.

2.   Honadle, Beth Walter. 2003. "The states' role in U.S. local government fiscal crises: A theoretical model and results of a national survey." *International Journal of Public Administration* 26 (13): 1431-1472.

3.   Coe, Charles K. 2008. "Preventing local government fiscal crises: Emerging best practices." *Public Administration Review* 68 (4): 759-767; Honadle, Beth Walter. 2003. "The states' role in U.S. local government fiscal crises: A theoretical model and results of a national survey." *International Journal of Public Administration* 26 (13): 1431-1472; Kloha, Philip, Carol S Weissert, and Robert Kleine. 2005. "Developing and testing a composite model to predict local fiscal distress." *Public Administration Review* 65 (3): 313-323.

4.   Scorsone, Eric A. 2014. Municipal Fiscal Emergency Laws: Background and Guide to State-Based Approaches. Working Paper 14-21. Washington, DC, Mercatus Center, George Mason University.

5. Honadle, Beth Walter. 2003. "The states' role in U.S. local government fiscal crises: A theoretical model and results of a national survey." *International Journal of Public Administration* 26 (13): 1431-1472.

6. Ibid.; Berman, David R. 1995. "Takeovers of local governments: An overview and evaluation of state policies." *Publius: The Journal of Federalism* 25 (3): 55-70; Cahill, Anthony G., Joseph A. James, Frank DeSanto, Richard Emmett, Thomas Hall, Bradley Horton, Ronald Seliga, Thomas Stoichess, Randall Stoner, and Dorrial Zurhellen. 1992. "Responding to Municipal Fiscal Distress: An Emerging Issue for State Governments in the 1990s." *Public Administration Review* 52 (1).

7. Ibid.

8. Ibid.

9. Ibid.

10. Honadle, Beth Walter. 2003. "The states' role in U.S. local government fiscal crises: A theoretical model and results of a national survey." *International Journal of Public Administration* 26 (13): 1431-1472

11. Ibid.; Cahill, Anthony G., Joseph A. James, Frank DeSanto, Richard Emmett, Thomas Hall, Bradley Horton, Ronald Seliga, Thomas Stoichess, Randall Stoner, and Dorrial Zurhellen. 1992. "Responding to Municipal Fiscal Distress: An Emerging Issue for State Governments in the 1990s." *Public Administration Review* 52 (1).

12. Honadle, Beth Walter. 2003. "The states' role in U.S. local government fiscal crises: A theoretical model and results of a national survey." *International Journal of Public Administration* 26 (13): 1431-1472.

13. Oosting, Jonathan, "Snyder signs replacement emergency manager law: We "heard, recognized and respected" will of voters." *MLive*, December 27, 2012. http://www.mlive.com/politics/index.ssf/2012/12/snyder_signs_replacement_emerg.html

14. Mallach, Alan, and Eric Scorsone. 2011. Long-Term Stress and Systemic Failure: Taking Seriously the Fiscal Crisis of America's Older Cities. Flint, MI: Center for Community Progress.

15. Ibid.

16. Scorsone, Eric, and Bateson, Nicolette, "Case Study: City of Flint, Michigan," East Lansing, MI: Michigan State University.

17. Ibid.

18. Mallach, Alan, and Eric Scorsone. 2011. Long-Term Stress and Systemic Failure: Taking Seriously the Fiscal Crisis of America's Older Cities. Flint, MI: Center for Community Progress.

19. City of Flint Comprehensive Annual Financial Report 2009-2015.

20. Mallach, Alan, and Eric Scorsone. 2011. Long-Term Stress and Systemic Failure: Taking Seriously the Fiscal Crisis of America's Older Cities. Flint, MI: Center for Community Progress.

21. Ibid.

22. Honadle, Beth Walter. 2003. "The states' role in U.S. local government fiscal crises: A theoretical model and results of a national survey." *International Journal of Public Administration* 26 (13): 1431-1472; Scorsone, Eric A. 2014. Municipal Fiscal Emergency Laws: Background and Guide to State-Based Approaches. Working Paper 14-21. Washington, DC, Mercatus Center, George Mason University; Skidmore, Mark, and Eric Scorsone. 2011. "Causes and consequences of fiscal stress in Michigan cities." *Regional Science and Urban Economics* 41 (4): 360-371.

23. City of Flint Comprehensive Annual Financial Report 2009-2015.

24. Associated Press, "Pontiac Silverdome sold at auction for $538,000," *New Orleans Business Review*, November 24, 2009.

25. Sterbenz, Christina, "How Flint, Michigan Became the Most Dangerous City in America." *Business Insider.* June 16, 2013. http://www.businessinsider.com/why-is-flint-michigan-dangerous-2013-6

26. Casserly, Meghan. 2012. "The Most Dangerous U.S. Cities For Women." *Forbes* (April, 26). Accessed April1, 2016.

27. City of Flint Comprehensive Annual Financial Report 2009-2015.

28. Fancher, Mark. 2012. Unelected and Unaccountable: Emergency Managers and Public Act 4's Threat to Representative Democracy. Detroit, MI: American Civil Liberties Union of Michigan.

29. Emergency Manager City of Flint Genesee County Michigan Order No. 2 Elimination of Salaries and Benefits of Mayor and City Council; Emergency Manager City of Flint Genesee County Michigan Order No. 5 Elimination of the Office of Ombudsman; Emergency Manager City of Flint Genesee County Michigan Order No. 6 Elimination of the Civil Service Commission; Emergency Manager City of Flint Genesee County Michigan Order No. 9 Mayor Dayne Walling's Responsibilities and Partial Restoration of Compensation.

30. Longley, Kristin, "Manager ousts several from Flint City Hall: council meetings, pay for members and Walling axed." *MLive* December 02, 2011. http://www.mlive.com/news/flint/index.ssf/2011/12/manager_ousts_seven_from_city.htm

31. Ibid.

32. Kimhi, Omer. 2010. "Chapter 9 of the Bankruptcy Code: A Solution in Search of a Problem." *Yale J. on Reg.* 27: 351.

33. Ibid.

34. Chung, Christine Sharlata. 2015. "Municipal Bankruptcy, Essential Municipal Services, and Taxpayers' Voice." *Widener LJ* 24: 43.

35. Ibid.

36. Knox, John, and John Levinson. 2009. *Municipal Bankruptcy: Avoiding and Using Chapter 9 in Times of Fiscal Stress.* New York, NY: Orrick, Herrington & Sutcliffe LLP.

37. Ibid.; Eucalitto, Cory, Kristen De Pena, and Shanan Younger. 2013. "Municipal Bankruptcy: An Overview for Local Officials." State Budget Solutions. Accessed May 17. http://www.statebudgetsolutions.org/publications/detail/municipal-bankruptcy-an-overview-for-local-officials.

38. Knox, John, and John Levinson. 2009. *Municipal Bankruptcy: Avoiding and Using Chapter 9 in Times of Fiscal Stress.* New York, NY: Orrick, Herrington & Sutcliffe LLP.

39. Kimhi, Omer. 2010. "Chapter 9 of the Bankruptcy Code: A Solution in Search of a Problem." *Yale J. on Reg.* 27: 351.

40. Chung, Christine Sharlata. 2015. "Municipal Bankruptcy, Essential Municipal Services, and Taxpayers' Voice." *Widener LJ* 24: 43.

CHAPTER 4

FLINT'S BUDGETARY CRISIS AND THE IMPACT ON PUBLIC HEALTH AND SAFETY

Jerry V. Graves, Alessandra Jerolleman
and Miriam Belblidia

Introduction

The State of Michigan's Public Act 72 allows the Governor to appoint an emergency manager to a local jurisdiction in the event of a fiscal emergency. In the case of Flint, the appointed emergency manager had a level of authority that exceeded that of the mayor and city council, and was responsible for making decisions that played a key role in the creation of the current water crisis. This failure to protect the public safety resulted in an Emergency Declaration, issued by the President under Title V of the Stafford Act, a largely unprecedented incident. Emergency Declarations are normally triggered by natural disasters, not by failures of local infrastructure. The scale of the Flint public health emergency triggered the declaration, allowing the Federal Government to provide direct assistance, an example being potable water. However, this raises key questions regarding the federal government's role in assisting local governments with infrastructure failures. Specifically, it raises questions about the federal government's role in emergency declarations and assistance following infrastructure failures that are a result of delayed maintenance, uninformed decision making, and lack of funding. The public administration failure in Flint extends beyond public health and fiscal considerations, into the underlying responsibility ensuring the safety of a government's citizens, responding to their concerns, and maintaining their trust.

This chapter addresses the challenges inherent in balancing fiscal constraints with public safety, particularly in the realm of water infrastructure, as well as key governance and policy issues related to water management, emergency management, and public health raised by the Flint Water Crisis. The chapter begins with a discussion of the nexus between water quality and public safety, followed by discussion of the water crisis in Flint, and ends with national implications for future consideration.

Water Quality and Public Safety

Safe drinking water is essential to public health and social prosperity in every community around the world.[1] However, the World Health Organization and the United Nations Children's Emergency Fund (UNICEF) Joint Monitoring Program estimate that 663 million people worldwide lack access to safe water.[2] Consequently, the production and distribution of safe water has become an increasingly prominent global public health concern over the past several decades.

A number of international treaties and organizations have confronted the challenges associated with the provision of safe water. Treaties such as the International Covenant on Civil and Political Rights have implied that safe drinking water should be considered a human right in participating states.[3] In fact, many states have recognized safe water as a human right either explicitly in their constitution or through precedents set via their judicial system.[4] The United Nations (UN) also formally declared in 2010 that access to "safe, acceptable, and affordable water" is a fundamental human right.[5] While the importance of safe water in the United States (U.S.) likewise cannot be overstated, a number of public policy and regulatory challenges persist at all levels of government.

The U.S. government has provided public drinking water-related services since the early 20th century. The U.S. Public Health Service (PHS) established the first potable water standards in 1914 for the purpose of curtailing the spread of communicable disease between states.[6] While there was no legal basis for the federal government to enforce water quality standards at the time, 14 states eventually adopted the PHS standards as guidelines for their public water systems.[7] The federal government did not actually begin regulating drinking water until Congress passed the Safe Drinking Water Act (SDWA) of 1974, which was proposed in response to growing public concerns following the release of two studies linking contaminated drinking water to cancer mortality (Quarles 1974, 69).[8] Congress has regularly amended and reauthorized the SDWA since its initial passage, and the legislation remains the centerpiece of U.S. public policy concerning the regulation of public water systems.

Regulatory Context

The SDWA requires the Environmental Protection Agency (EPA) to engage in source water protection activities, monitor water treatment and distribution systems, and share information with the public regarding water quality (EPA 2015).[9] In accordance with the SDWA, the EPA is also charged with identifying and studying specific potential contaminants and setting Maximum Contaminant Levels (MCL) for public water systems.[10] The greatest challenge associated with the SDWA is that while the EPA is charged with establishing drinking water standards, individual states are ultimately responsible for monitoring and enforcement of over 160,000 public water systems nationwide (Cory & Rahman 2009, 1827).[11]

As per the SDWA, most states have *primacy* with respect to EPA standards, meaning that states are legally responsible for enforcement at the local level.[12] A condition of primacy is that states agree to implement standards in their respective jurisdictions that are equal to or more stringent than EPA standards.[13] Issues relative to state primacy and the perception of SDWA as a largely unfunded federal mandate have hindered the legislation throughout its existence.[14] This dynamic has perpetuated a situation in which: (1) funding for local public water system repairs, maintenance, and improvements is lacking, particularly in less affluent communities; (2) the states' financial and administrative capacity to enforce EPA standards is sometimes compromised; and (3) the EPA is often burdened with taking SWDA enforcement actions against states.[15]

EPA standards regarding the use of lead materials in public water system components have also been problematic. Congress amended the SDWA in 1986 to include a ban on all water system materials that were not considered "lead-free" (pipes containing no more than 8% lead and solder or flux containing no more than .2% lead).[16] The SDWA was further amended in 1988 to include the Lead Contamination Control Act, which required the EPA to monitor water coolers containing lead materials and provide guidance on managing lead contamination in drinking water supplies at schools.[17]

Since EPA regulations regarding lead did not have the effect of completely banning all lead fixtures, the possibility of lead contamination in drinking water still existed despite the 1986 and 1988 amendments to the SDWA. The EPA subsequently published the Lead and Copper Rule in 1991. This measure required local system monitoring at consumer taps and established lead limits of 15 parts per billion (ppb) and copper limits of 1.3 parts per million (ppm).[18] Exceedance of the established limits at 10% or more of the local sample sites now triggers public notification of health threats and corrosion control measures for the water source.[19] The purpose of the corrosion control provision was to protect the water source from causing lead to leach into the water supply when lead fixtures in the system became wetted. The EPA has amended the Lead and Copper Rule several times following the rule's initial publishing.

Congress also continued to amend the SDWA in order to further regulate lead fixtures and lead content in public drinking water systems. A set of 1996 amendments to the SDWA included a ban on the use of plumbing fixtures that were not considered lead-free.[20] Finally, Congress passed the Reduction of Lead in Drinking Water Act of 2011, which reduced the required threshold for lead-free materials and exempted certain non-potable water fixtures from the lead-free standard.[21] As with many other provisions of the SDWA, the enforcement of lead standards has proven challenging due to a lack of resources, monitoring, and oversight at all levels of government.[22]

Overall, the standards established for safe drinking water in accordance with the SDWA have been critical to the provision of safe drinking water in the U.S. But the financial and administrative challenges associated with the states' primacy in enforcing the standards set forth by the EPA have caused lapses in the provision of safe drinking water, and in some instances, public health crises. Lead is just one example of the many SDWA regulatory challenges faced by the EPA, states, and public water system operators in the U.S. Aging public water system infrastructure and diminishing public resources are perhaps the greatest threats to the provision of safe drinking water in the U.S. going forward.[23]

Infrastructure

The performance of public water systems typically depends on the functionality of four key system components: (1) water source; (2) physical infrastructure; (3) administrative infrastructure (capacity to operate, monitor, and maintain); and (4) public policy and regulations (standards, support, and funding).[24] Sourcing fresh water will continue to be a concern into the 21st century as water resources are depleted at an ever-increasing rate.[25] Public policy, regulations, and the associated administrative challenges relative to the provision of drinking water in the U.S. have already been summarized in the preceding section. However, the condition and performance of the physical drinking water system infrastructure in the U.S. are worthy of further discussion.

The challenges associated with funding public water system infrastructure repairs and improvements in the US have been well documented.[26] The EPA has projected that short-term (2011-2030) public water system infrastructure capital improvement needs will cost over $384 billion nationwide.[27] This figure represents a dramatic increase from the EPA's 1999 projection of $225 billion (adjusted for inflation as of January 2011).[28] Similarly, the American Society of Civil Engineers (ASCE) assigned drinking water infrastructure a "D" grade in the organization's 2013 Report Card for America's Infrastructure.[29] This grade was a reflection of ASCE's opinion that very little had changed since 2009, when the organization also assigned drinking water infrastructure a grade of "D."[30] The ASCE has projected that meeting short-term (2013-2033) public water system infrastructure needs will cost nearly $335 billion nationwide.[31]

Maintaining functional public water systems that comply with the SDWA has become an increasingly expensive endeavor for municipalities. The cost of compliance has outpaced the local resources available for system maintenance and improvements, as reflected by the current drinking water infrastructure needs identified by the EPA and ASCE.[32] In response to this paradox, Congress included provisions for a Drinking Water State Revolving Fund (DWSRF) when it amended the SDWA in 1996.[33] The DWSRF essentially functions as a federal-state partnership that provides a mechanism for various types of financial assistance, which can be used for certain public water system infrastructure projects involving one or more of the following: (1) treatment; (2) transmission and distribution; (3) source; (4) storage; (5) consolidation; and (6) creation of new systems.[34] Although the DWSRF facilitated $17.3 billion in federal assistance and leveraged $27.9 billion in state funding between 1996 and 2014, total DSWRF expenditures (roughly $45 billion as of 2014) have covered only a fraction of projected needs.[35] It is clear that federal and state subsidies alone will not solve the drinking water infrastructure crisis in the U.S.[36] Unfortunately, many municipalities find themselves in financial positions that are not conducive to largescale capital investment.

Despite the DSWRF funding opportunities afforded in many states, the level of capital improvement expenditures required to address public water system infrastructure needs in the U.S. remains well beyond the financial capacity of local governments.[37] In fact, many municipalities can hardly even afford to maintain their public water system infrastructure at levels that comply with federal and state standards.[38] Shrinking cities such as Flint, Michigan have a particularly difficult time funding capital improvements considering that the costs associated with their drinking water systems are generally fixed; the systems themselves are not flexible or scalable, and any improvements must be at least partially funded by a declining population and tax base (Herz, 2006).[39] The increasing cost of public water system improvements and the continued decline in city populations also exponentially increase the per capita cost of needed improvements, and make safe drinking water even more unaffordable for remaining residents.[40]

Emergency Financial Managers and Emergency Managers

The media coverage of the Flint Water Crisis has led to confusion regarding the role of the appointed Emergency Financial Managers. This was largely due to its 2012 abbreviation to Emergency Manager, a title already used in most communities. An Emergency Manager, in the traditional sense, is responsible for ensuring that a community is prepared for and able to respond to natural and man-made emergencies. Emergency Financial Managers, on the other hand, are in place to make financial decisions on behalf of jurisdictions that are in extreme financial distress. Michigan's financial Emergency Manager legislation was passed under Public Act 72 in 1990, authorizing the state to intervene in local governments experiencing financial emergencies.

Although the difference between an Emergency Financial Manager appointed by the state to handle financial emergencies and an Emergency Manager tasked with protecting communities from natural and man-made emergencies appears clear cut, the general public does not always fully understand these roles, and the emergency management community has faced increasing questions about water quality over the past year (Holdeman, 2016).[41] Emergency management does provide a framework that can be useful for the management of financial emergencies by using the concept of a cycle, which includes mitigation, preparedness, response, and recovery. According to Kasdan, local jurisdictions could minimize the impacts of fiscal insolvency by identifying and acknowledging the impending crisis before it occurs, as opposed to simply responding with last minute state interventions.[42] In other words, they could choose to invest in preparedness and mitigation in order to reduce response and recovery costs. He notes that the fiscal crisis has led to an increase in state interventions, with varied results, and suggests that a warning system based on local indicators is needed.

In 2014, an article in the *Journal of the American Water Works Association* identified the need for better Consequence Management Procedures for community water systems in the event of a water quality event. The authors called for the creation of Standard Operating Procedures and a plan for informing the public. This type of detailed response strategy is completely within the purview of traditional emergency management and may be an area in which emergency managers can play a role—even if only as advisors to the creation of emergency plans for water systems.

Flint Water Crisis

The Flint Water Crisis exemplifies the challenges of providing safe drinking water in the United States. A complex regulatory framework and unfunded mandates, in combination with local tax bases too poor to maintain or upgrade aging infrastructure, as well as lax oversight and decisions based primarily on cost savings, have resulted in a public health crisis. While the situation in Flint is ongoing and the full impact remains to be determined, these challenges are not isolated to Flint. The crisis in Flint is considered the second worst drinking water emergency documented in United States history after the 1993 Cryptosporidium outbreak in Milwaukee, Wisconsin.[43] It is important to note that localities throughout the U.S. are experiencing similar, less-publicized crises, and that the potential for future crises grows as infrastructure ages.[44]

Historical Context

Flint, Michigan's history is inextricably linked with the rise of the automobile industry in the United States. General Motors (GM) selected Flint as its corporate headquarters in 1908 and opened its Flint Assembly plant in 1947.[45] In doing so, GM became a driving force in the local economy.

In the decades following WWII, GM's corporate strategy focused on investment in suburban manufacturing centers, including the construction of eight additional manufacturing centers in Genesee County, where the city of Flint is located.[46] This strategy shifted resources and jobs away from Flint, blurring local boundaries and leading to political divisions. Efforts were made in the 1950s to expand Flint's boundaries and push for regional government; dubbed the "New Flint" proposal, this effort ultimately failed in large part due to white, suburban opposition.[47] African American residents were also dubious of "New Flint," having been excluded from the coalition responsible for the proposal, and due to concerns that a regional approach towards governance would disenfranchise African American voters.[48] Unfortunately, the defeat of the "New Flint" proposal heralded the gradual loss of Flint's higher-income tax base, which eventually contributed to lessened investments in necessary infrastructure. The loss of this infrastructure funding led directly to the disintegration of drinking water infrastructure, and ultimately to the water crisis itself.

As GM continued to invest in the suburbs of Genesee County, GM plant managers were able to successfully lobby elected Flint officials for the extension of necessary water and sewer lines for industrial production to seven of their new suburban plants.[49] Decades later, when GM discovered that the Flint water supply was corroding engines manufactured in the Genesee plants, they received permission from Flint's emergency manager to disconnect from Flint's water supply. This request came a full year before Flint's residents were urged by city officials to stop drinking the municipal water.[50]

Despite the move from urban to suburban manufacturing facilities, the auto industry continued to provide reliable jobs to Flint residents. As a result, population of Flint grew steadily between 1940 and 1960. However, deindustrialization eventually shifted production overseas and by the 1980s, GM had closed two plants in Flint and laid off a total of 29,000 workers across four states.[51] The population of Flint dropped, resulting in tax revenues insufficient for the funding of infrastructure maintenance, which was originally built to support a much larger and better employed population.[52]

As economic forces were pushing automobile production overseas, federal housing policies in the U.S. simultaneously encouraged the growth of suburbs and white flight. White residents of Flint were able to relocate to the suburbs, enabled by racist housing policies that subsidized these moves, while redlining, a practice of denying loans within certain neighborhoods, prevented lending within African American neighborhoods.[53] This further eroded the local tax base in many cities, including Flint. By 2015, 40.1% of Flint residents were living in poverty. According to the U.S. Census, the median household income between 2010-2014 was $24,679.

The housing and economic crisis in the early 2000s further affected Flint's tax base. The recession's impact on housing prices is expected to have long lasting effects on local government finance.[54] Skidmore and Scorscone's analysis of expenditure patterns in Michigan cities between 2005-2009 found that "expenditures in the General Government, Public Works, and Parks and Recreation categories were responsive to fiscal stress, and Capital Expenditures have been particularly vulnerable." While this analysis stated that expenditures for essential services such as Public Safety are generally not affected, this does not take into account the direct correlation between public works expenditures and safety. Instead, it presents a limited view of safety that is based upon expenditures for fire and police.

Other researchers have also found that less visible infrastructure, such as water and wastewater systems, receive even less investment than more visible systems such as roads and bridges due to a lack of public awareness.[55] In their research on water and wastewater management in shrinking cities, which included a case study of Flint, Faust et al. found that the per capita costs of systems increase as population declines and that income inequalities leave many customers unable to afford the increased rates. Additionally, many jurisdictions respond to budget crises by cutting personnel, something that further exacerbates maintenance challenges and threatens public safety. Flint presents a clear case study on how economic impacts led to costly fiscal decisions that undermined public safety.

Public Act 72, passed in 1990 in Michigan, authorizes the state to intervene when local government is facing a financial emergency. This intervention can include the appointment of an Emergency Financial Manager (pre-2012) or Emergency Manager (post-2012) who is given some control of local financial decisions on behalf of the state.[56] Since 2011, 17 municipalities and school districts have had an appointed Emergency Financial Manager or Emergency Manager.[57] The approaches taken by appointed Emergency Financial Managers and Emergency Managers in Michigan have ranged from efforts to work with local leaders to strict financial receivership.

The City of Flint had four different Emergency Financial Managers or Emergency Managers over four years, two of whom were involved with key decisions that led to the water crisis.[58] However, although there is a clear correlation between the fiscal crisis in Flint and the local decision to switch water supplies to the Flint River, the collapse of government oversight at the state level is more directly responsible for the public health crisis—the

Michigan Department of Environmental Quality (MDEQ) had the regulatory authority and did not exercise it. The decision to take water from the Flint River would not have proved disastrous if appropriate corrosion control had been put in place. Corrosive controls, including chemicals such as phosphoric acid used to reduce corrosion, would have been more costly; however, the cost of these preventative measures would have been incomparable—in terms of financial and health impacts—to the cost of the resulting crisis.

MDEQ failed to require additional corrosion control when the City of Flint switched from the Detroit to the Flint River in 2014, and proceeded to ignore complaints by residents of Flint, who had begun reporting poor water quality by 2015.[59] The agency is accused of hiding test results and failing to act in the face of an emerging public health emergency.[60] The culture of minimal compliance at MDEQ contributed to this crisis, as did extensive state budget cuts that significantly curtailed the regulatory abilities of the agency.[61] The Attorney General has pressed involuntary manslaughter charges against several public officials involved, but no trials have gone to court as of yet.[62]

Table 1. Timeline of Events

Date	Action
2011	Flint brought under control of Emergency Manager for financial oversight.
March 25, 2013	Flint's Mayor and City Council approve switching city's water source from Detroit to the Karegnondi Water Authority (KWA), which uses Flint River water
March 29, 2013	Council's affirmative vote was supported and signed as an Executive Order by then-Emergency Manager Edward Kurtz
April 2014	Flint switches water source from Detroit to Flint River, without corrosion control treatment.
October 2014	General Motors receives permission from Flint's emergency manager to switch back to Detroit water after realizing that the Flint River Water was corroding the engines at its plants.

March 2015	Flint City Council votes to identify a means of returning to Detroit's water, but are prevented from doing so by the current Emergency Manager, Jerry Ambrose (*Mother Jones* 2016).
October 1, 2015	City officials urge Flint residents to stop drinking the water.
October 16, 2015	Flint reconnects to Detroit's water and advises residents not to use unfiltered tap water.
October 2015	The Michigan Department of Environmental Quality (MDEQ) announces that it had followed the wrong monitoring protocol for Flint. Reportedly, the city conducted water testing incorrectly.
November 2015	EPA clarifies corrosion control requirements for large systems that previously purchased treated water.
January 2016	The city and the governor of Michigan each declare a state of emergency. President Obama issues an emergency declaration on January 16, 2016, under the Stafford Act.
January 21, 2016	The Environmental Protection Agency (EPA) issues an emergency order directing the city and state to take immediate actions to address concerns over the city's water system. Requirements include corrosion control, posting online lead monitoring results and weekly reports, and ensuring the city's capacity to operate the system in compliance with federal regulations.
February 1, 2016	EPA administrator, Susan Hedman, whose region includes Flint, Michigan, resigns over the agency's response to the water crisis.
February 4, 2016	H.R. 4479 - Families of Flint Act introduced in Congress, which would authorize infrastructure grants, increase DWSRF loan forgiveness, provide grants under federal health, education, and nutrition programs, and establish the Center on Excellence on Lead Exposure.

Public Health Impacts

The toxicity of lead has been well documented, as it has the ability to affect the neurologic, hematologic, gastrointestinal, cardiovascular, and renal systems.[63] Children can be particularly susceptible to negative health effects when excessive levels of lead are found in the water supply; children in Flint were found to have elevated blood-lead levels during the period in which the city switched to the Flint River water supply.[64]

Young children and pregnant women are most affected by lead. In young children, especially those under five years of age, lead impacts the developing nervous system and has been linked with lower intelligence quotient (IQ), attention deficit disorder (ADD), and aggression.[65] In pregnant women, lead has been linked with miscarriage, stillbirth, premature birth and low birth weight, as well as minor malformations.[66]

According to the World Health Organization, "acute exposures to lead may cause gastrointestinal disturbances (anorexia, nausea, vomiting, abdominal pain), hepatic and renal damage, hypertension and neurological effects (malaise, drowsiness, encephalopathy) that may lead to convulsions and death." Local doctors in Flint began reporting signs among their patients within months of switching water supplies in 2014, including rashes and hair loss.[67]

The full and long-term consequences of elevated lead levels in Flint residents, caused by the government's decision to switch water supplies, remains to be seen. However, given the established links between lead and its short and long term, this public health crisis will have a lasting effect on the population in Flint. Efforts to redress the impact of lead contamination in the water supply may include an increased need for health care spending and special education services; moreover, the erosion of public trust in government will take much longer to repair.

National Implications and Policy Questions Raised

Deficiencies in U.S. public infrastructure, including drinking water and in virtually every other category, have been well documented.[68] The crisis in Flint provides an unfortunate illustration of what many had long feared: that deteriorating, aging public infrastructure would someday directly result in a major public health and safety crisis. There are several on-going public health emergencies across the country, as various cities wrestle with again public infrastructure, but none that have generated the level of media attention that Flint has seen.[69] The Flint water crisis presents an opportunity for the nation to identify long-term solutions to this problem and restore public trust.

The crisis in Flint also highlights the challenges associated with the federal model of SDWA enforcement and state primacy. As states also struggle with budget cuts, their ability to ensure regulatory compliance becomes further curtailed. Additionally, when local decisions are being made by state representatives there are conflicts of interest as the state is forced to regulate its own actions without any outside oversight.

Given that the crisis occurred in a shrinking city during a time in which a state-appointed Emergency Manager was in charge of local affairs, there are other serious national implications relative to environmental justice and democracy. A number of specific policy questions may be gleaned from this sweeping set of national implications. For instance, is an external Emergency Manager more likely to take long-term risks to show short-term savings? On the other hand, local politicians are often accused of taking just that approach.

Entities such as the ASCE and EPA have documented the poor condition of water infrastructure in the U.S. and estimated that addressing current needs would cost between $335 and $384 billion.[70] Although the DWSRF has resulted in approximately $45 billion in water infrastructure investment since 1996, this level of federal and state funding alone will not sufficiently address the overwhelming (and constantly growing) water infrastructure needs in the U.S.[71] Local capacity to fund water infrastructure needs has also been diminishing, particularly in shrinking cities such as Flint. How will water infrastructure improvements be funded going forward? Should the Federal Government play a larger role in funding needed improvements in the most at-risk communities, such as shrinking cities?

Concerns regarding the federal nature of EPA standard-setting and state primacy have existed since the SDWA was first passed in 1974. The Flint crisis punctuated the validity of these long-held concerns, as evidenced by the timeline of events and resulting aftermath. These events included congressional hearings in which public officials such as the EPA Administrator, EPA Regional Administrator (who resigned as a result of the crisis), Governor of Michigan, state-appointed Emergency Manager (formerly referred to as an Emergency Financial Manager), and former Mayor of Flint were questioned regarding their role in the decision to use the Flint River as a water source without engaging in the appropriate corrosion control measures. The Flint scenario was obviously further complicated and is somewhat unique due to the involvement of the Emergency Manager. However, the policy question remains: does the SDWA provide the sufficient administrative framework and resources for the effective enforcement of drinking water standards? Additionally, is state primacy the most effective means of SDWA enforcement?

The legal impetus for the state-appointment of Emergency Financial Managers in Michigan and elsewhere is that the state must intervene when a local entity cannot manage its own financial affairs. Such intervention is typically triggered by a declaration of bankruptcy on the part of the local entity, and the Emergency Financial Manager's sole purpose is to make decisions that will ensure the future solvency of the local entity being managed. However, the Flint crisis has demonstrated that decisions made during times of state-appointed emergency management must go beyond finances alone and that Emergency Financial Managers should ensure that public health and safety concerns are given appropriate consideration. This is a particularly sensitive issue when one considers how decisions made by the Emergency Financial Manager have resulted in grave public health consequences in the city of Flint, as well as irreversible health consequences for individuals who were repeatedly exposed to the toxic water. Should the legal provisions for emergency management in Michigan and elsewhere appropriately account for public health and safety considerations? Do the legal provisions for emergency management appropriately provide for continued local participation in decision-making during times of emergency management?

A final policy issue raised is just how much of a role the profession of emergency management can play in the face of failing infrastructure. Many Emergency Operations Plans and Hazard Mitigation Plans address public health and infrastructure, but they rely heavily on their partners to ensure that the systems are fully functional during normal operations. Some of the resiliency frameworks, such as that being used by the Rockefeller Foundation's *100 Resilient Cities* initiative, do address pervasive infrastructure challenges through the frame of stressors on the broader system—but it is unclear how best to resolve these challenges.[72] Perhaps emergency management as a profession can contribute solutions to these challenges. Further research and dialogue are needed in order to identify the best collaborative solutions.

Conclusion

The Flint Water Crisis represents the culmination of several phenomena that are occurring across urban America, including the shrinking footprint of cities and the inability or unwillingness of municipalities to invest in repairing or otherwise improving aging public infrastructure. Although the importance of clean and safe water is well understood around the world, public health and safety concerns in Flint were somehow overlooked when the decision was made to utilize the Flint River as a water source without engaging in the appropriate corrosion control measures and under a resource-constrained environment. That such a decision was made while Flint was in receivership and under the control of a state-appointed Emergency Manager. This calls into question not only the effectiveness of state primacy in the enforcement of the SDWA, but also whether the concept of receivership is too myopic and should be revisited. Public health must remain the top priority, above and beyond budget shortfalls and short-term political solutions. Flint may have served as a reminder of this, or it may simply be the first of many crises to come.

Notes

1. Paul, Tara. "Plugging the Democracy Drain in the Struggle for Universal Access to Safe Drinking Water," *Indiana Journal of Global Legal Studies*: Vol. 20 (2013): Issue 1, Article 16.

2. UNICEF. Water and Hygiene Introduction. 2015. Accessed April 12, 2016. http://www.unicef.org/wash/index_3951.html.

3. Paul, Tara. "Plugging the Democracy Drain in the Struggle for Universal Access to Safe Drinking Water," *Indiana Journal of Global Legal Studies*: Vol. 20 (2013): Issue 1, Article 16.

4. Ibid.

5. UN. International Decade for Action. 2010. Accessed April 12, 2016. http://www.un.org/waterforlifedecade/human_right_to_water.shtml.

6. Kyros, P. N. (1974). Legislative History of the Safe Drinking Water Act. *Journal-American Water Works Association*, 66 (10): 566-569.

7. Wiant, D., Vanderstraeten, C., Maurer, J., Pursley, J., Terrell, J., & Sintay, B. J. (2014). On the validity of density overrides for VMAT lung SBRT plan-

ning. *Medical physics*, 41 (8Part1); Kyros, P. N. (1974). Legislative History of the Safe Drinking Water Act. *Journal-American Water Works Association*, 66 (10): 566-569.

8. Quarles, H. D., Hanawalt, R. B., & Odum, W. E. (1974). Lead in Small Mammals, Plants, and Soil at Varying Distances from a Highway. *Journal of Applied Ecology*, 11 (3): 937-949; Trager, S. M., Hawkins, R. C., Staples, M. A., & McKenney, L. B. (1994). Safe Drinking Water Act reauthorization: In the eye of the storm. *Natural Resources & Environment*, 9 (1): 17-55.

9. EPA. Summary of the Safe Drinking Water Act. October 8, 2015. Accessed April 12, 2016. https://www.epa.gov/laws-regulations/summary-safe-drinking-water-act.; Trager, S. M., Hawkins, R. C., Staples, M. A., & McKenney, L. B. (1994). Safe Drinking Water Act reauthorization: In the eye of the storm. *Natural Resources & Environment*, 9 (1): 17-55.

10. Grooms, K. K. (2016). Does water quality improve when a Safe Drinking Water Act violation is issued? A study of the effectiveness of the SDWA in California. *The BE Journal of Economic Analysis & Policy*, 16 (1): 1-23.

11. Wiant, D., Vanderstraeten, C., Maurer, J., Pursley, J., Terrell, J., & Sintay, B. J. (2014). On the validity of density overrides for VMAT lung SBRT planning. *Medical physics*, 41 (8Part1); Cory, Dennis C. and Tauhidur Rahman. "Environmental justice and enforcement of the safe drinking water act: The Arizona arsenic experience." *Ecological Economics*, Vol. 68 (2009): 1827.

12. Trager, S. M., Hawkins, R. C., Staples, M. A., & McKenney, L. B. (1994). Safe Drinking Water Act reauthorization: In the eye of the storm. *Natural Resources & Environment*, 9 (1): 17-55.

13. Cory, Dennis C. and Tauhidur Rahman. "Environmental justice and enforcement of the safe drinking water act: The Arizona arsenic experience." *Ecological Economics*, Vol. 68 (2009): 1829.

14. United States. Congressional Research Service. Lead in Flint, Michigan's Drinking Water: Federal Regulatory Role. By Mary Tiemann. March 2, 2016. Accessed March 15, 2016. https://www.fas.org/sgp/crs/misc/IN10446.pdf; Faust, Kasey M., Dulcy M. Abraham, and Shawn P. McElmurry. "Water and Wastewater Infrastructure Management in Shrinking Cities." *Public Works Management & Policy* (2015): 1-29. Accessed January 1, 2016. EBSCO.; Daley, D. M., Mullin, M., & Rubado, M. E. (2013). State Agency Discretion in a Delegated Federal Program: Evidence from Drinking Water Investment. *Publius: The Journal of Federalism*, 44 (4): 564-586; Trager, S. M., Hawkins, R. C., Staples, M. A., & McKenney, L. B. (1994). Safe Drinking Water Act reauthorization: In the eye of the storm. *Natural Resources & Environment*, 9 (1): 17-55.

15. Daley, D. M., Mullin, M., & Rubado, M. E. (2013). State Agency Discretion in a Delegated Federal Program: Evidence from Drinking Water Investment. *Publius: The Journal of Federalism, 44* (4): 564-586; Cory, Dennis C. and Tauhidur Rahman. "Environmental justice and enforcement of the safe drinking water act: The Arizona arsenic experience." *Ecological Economics*, Vol. 68 (2009): 1825-1837; Levin, Ronnie B., Paul R. Epstein, Tim E. Ford, Winston Harrington, Erik Olson, and Eric G. Reichard. "U.S. Drinking Water Challenges in the Twenty-First Century." *Environmental Health Perspectives* 110, no. S1 (February 01, 2002): 43-52. Accessed January 1, 2016. doi:10.1289/ehp.02110s143; Trager, S. M., Hawkins, R. C., Staples, M. A., & McKenney, L. B. (1994). Safe Drinking Water Act reauthorization: In the eye of the storm. *Natural Resources & Environment, 9* (1): 17-55.

16. EPA. Summary of the Safe Drinking Water Act. October 8, 2015. Accessed April 12, 2016. https://www.epa.gov/laws-regulations/summary-safe-drinking-water-act.

17. Advocacy and Public Policymaking. Accessed April 12, 2016. http://lobby.la.psu.edu/

18. EPA. Drinking Water Infrastructure Needs Assessment and Survey: Fifth Report to Congress. 2011. Accessed April 12, 2016. https://www.epa.gov/sites/production/files/2015-07/documents/epa816r13006.pdf

19. Ibid.

20. EPA. Summary of the Safe Drinking Water Act. October 8, 2015. Accessed April 12, 2016. https://www.epa.gov/laws-regulations/summary-safe-drinking-water-act.

21. Ibid.

22. United States. Congressional Research Service. Lead in Flint, Michigan's Drinking Water: Federal Regulatory Role. By Mary Tiemann. March 2, 2016. Accessed March 15, 2016. https://www.fas.org/sgp/crs/misc/IN10446.pdf: 1.

23. Cotruvo, Joseph A. "The Safe Drinking Water Act: Current and Future." *American Water Works Association*, Vol. 104, No. 1, Infrastructure (January 2012): 57-62.

24. Vanderslice, James. "Drinking Water Infrastructure and Environmental Disparities: Evidence and Methodological Considerations." *American Journal of Public Health* 101, no. S1 (2011): 109. Accessed January 1, 2016. doi:10.2105/ajph.2011.300189.

25. Levin, Ronnie B., Paul R. Epstein, Tim E. Ford, Winston Harrington, Erik Olson, and Eric G. Reichard. "U.S. Drinking Water Challenges in the Twenty-First

Century." *Environmental Health Perspectives* 110, no. S1 (February 01, 2002): 43. Accessed January 1, 2016. doi:10.1289/ehp.02110s143.

26. Faust, Kasey M., Dulcy M. Abraham, and Shawn P. McElmurry. "Water and Wastewater Infrastructure Management in Shrinking Cities." *Public Works Management & Policy*, 2015, 1-29. Accessed January 1, 2016. EBSCO; Daley, D. M., Mullin, M., & Rubado, M. E. (2013). "State Agency Discretion in a Delegated Federal Program: Evidence from Drinking Water Investment." *Publius: The Journal of Federalism*, 44 (4): 564-586; Paul, Tara. "Plugging the Democracy Drain in the Struggle for Universal Access to Safe Drinking Water," *Indiana Journal of Global Legal Studies*: Vol. 20 (2013): Issue 1, Article 16; Cotruvo, Joseph A. "The Safe Drinking Water Act: Current and Future." *American Water Works Association*, Vol. 104, No. 1, Infrastructure (January 2012): 57-62; EPA. Drinking Water Infrastructure Needs Assessment and Survey: Fifth Report to Congress. 2011. Accessed April 12, 2016. https://www.epa.gov/sites/production/files/2015-07/documents/epa816r13006.pdf; Baird, Gregory M. "Money Matters: The Silver Bullet for Aging Water Distribution System?" *American Water Works Association Journal* 103, no. 6 (June 2011): 14-23. Accessed January 1, 2016. EBSCO; Cory, Dennis C. and Tauhidur Rahman. "Environmental justice and enforcement of the safe drinking water act: The Arizona arsenic experience." *Ecological Economics*, Vol. 68 (2009): 1825-1837; Levin, Ronnie B., Paul R. Epstein, Tim E. Ford, Winston Harrington, Erik Olson, and Eric G. Reichard. "U.S. Drinking Water Challenges in the Twenty-First Century." *Environmental Health Perspectives* 110, no. S1 (February 01, 2002): 43-52. Accessed January 1, 2016. doi:10.1289/ehp.02110s143; Trager, S. M., Hawkins, R. C., Staples, M. A., & McKenney, L. B. (1994). Safe Drinking Water Act reauthorization: In the eye of the storm. *Natural Resources & Environment, 9* (1): 17-55.

27. EPA. Drinking Water Infrastructure Needs Assessment and Survey: Fifth Report to Congress. 2011. Accessed April 12, 2016. https://www.epa.gov/sites/production/files/2015-07/documents/epa816r13006.pdf.

28. Ibid.; Levin, Ronnie B., Paul R. Epstein, Tim E. Ford, Winston Harrington, Erik Olson, and Eric G. Reichard. "U.S. Drinking Water Challenges in the Twenty-First Century." *Environmental Health Perspectives* 110, no. S1 (February 01, 2002): 43. Accessed January 1, 2016. doi:10.1289/ehp.02110s143.

29. ASCE. Report Card for America's Infrastructure. 2013. Accessed April 12, 2016. http://www.infrastructurereportcard.org/

30. Paul, Tara. "Plugging the Democracy Drain in the Struggle for Universal Access to Safe Drinking Water," *Indiana Journal of Global Legal Studies*: Vol. 20 (2013): Issue 1, Article 16.

31. ASCE. Report Card for America's Infrastructure. 2013. Accessed April 12, 2016. http://www.infrastructurereportcard.org/.

32. Paul, Tara. "Plugging the Democracy Drain in the Struggle for Universal Access to Safe Drinking Water," *Indiana Journal of Global Legal Studies*: Vol. 20 (2013): 471. Issue 1, Article 16.

33. Daley, D. M., Mullin, M., & Rubado, M. E. (2013). State Agency Discretion in a Delegated Federal Program: Evidence from Drinking Water Investment. *Publius: The Journal of Federalism*, 44 (4): 564-586.

34. EPA. Summary of the Safe Drinking Water Act. October 8, 2015. Accessed April 12, 2016. https://www.epa.gov/laws-regulations/summary-safe-drinking-water-act.

35. Ibid.; ASCE. Report Card for America's Infrastructure. 2013. Accessed April 12, 2016. http://www.infrastructurereportcard.org/; EPA. Drinking Water Infrastructure Needs Assessment and Survey: Fifth Report to Congress. 2011. Accessed April 12, 2016. https://www.epa.gov/sites/production/files/2015-07/documents/epa816r13006.pdf.

36. Levin, Ronnie B., Paul R. Epstein, Tim E. Ford, Winston Harrington, Erik Olson, and Eric G. Reichard. "U.S. Drinking Water Challenges in the Twenty-First Century." *Environmental Health Perspectives* 110, no. S1 (February 01, 2002): 43-52. Accessed January 1, 2016. doi:10.1289/ehp.02110s143.

37. Paul, Tara. "Plugging the Democracy Drain in the Struggle for Universal Access to Safe Drinking Water," *Indiana Journal of Global Legal Studies*: Vol. 20 (2013): 471. Issue 1, Article 16.

38. Faust, Kasey M., Dulcy M. Abraham, and Shawn P. McElmurry. "Water and Wastewater Infrastructure Management in Shrinking Cities." *Public Works Management & Policy*, 2015, 7. Accessed January 1, 2016. EBSCO.

39. Herz, R. (2006). "Buried infrastructure in shrinking cities," *International Symposium: Coping with City Shrinkage and Demographic Change - Lessons from Around the Globe*; Hummel, D., & Lux, A. (2007). Population decline and infrastructure: The case of the German water supply system. *Vienna Yearbook of Population Research*, 167-191; Schlor, H., Hake, J. F., & Kuckshinrichs, H. (2009). Demographics as a new challenge for sustainable development in the German wastewater sector. *International Journal of Environmental Technology and Management*, 10 (3-4): 327-352.

40. Faust, Kasey M., Dulcy M. Abraham, and Shawn P. McElmurry. "Water and Wastewater Infrastructure Management in Shrinking Cities." *Public Works Management & Policy*, 2015, 6. Accessed January 1, 2016. EBSCO.

41. Holdeman, Eric. (March 21, 2016). "'Real'" Emergency Managers Don't Like Michigan's Use of the Term." Retrieved from: http://www.govtech.com/em/

emergency-blogs/disaster-zone/real-emergency-managers-dont-like-michi
gans-use-of-the-term.html

42. Kasdan, David O. "Emergency Management 2.0: This Time, It's Financial."
    Urban Affairs Review, 2015, 1-19. Accessed March 1, 2016. doi:10.1177/10
    78087415574730.

43. Kozacek, Codi. "Michigan DEQ's Responsibility to Ensure Public Safety Col-
    lapsed in Flint." RSS. January 25, 2016. Accessed February 03, 2016. http://
    www.resilience.org/stories/2016-01-25/michigan-deq-s-responsibility-to-en
    sure-public-safety-collapsed-in-flint.

44. Weesjes, Elke. "Flint Crisis Hasn't Steeled the Nation Against the Health Risks
    of Lead." *Natural Hazards Observer*. March 2016.

45. "Welcome to Flint." Flint Assembly. Accessed April 29, 2016. http://flintassem
    bly.gm.com.

46. Highsmith, Andrew R. "Beyond Corporate Abandonment: General Motors
    and the Politics of Metropolitan Capitalism in Flint, Michigan." *Journal of Ur-
    ban History* 40, no. 1 (2014): 31-47. Accessed January 1, 2016. EBSCO.

47. Highsmith, Andrew R. "Beyond Corporate Abandonment: General Motors
    and the Politics of Metropolitan Capitalism in Flint, Michigan." *Journal of Ur-
    ban History* 40, no. 1 (2014): 32. Accessed January 1, 2016. EBSCO.

48. Highsmith, Andrew R. "Beyond Corporate Abandonment: General Motors
    and the Politics of Metropolitan Capitalism in Flint, Michigan." *Journal of Ur-
    ban History* 40, no. 1 (2014): 40. Accessed January 1, 2016. EBSCO.

49. Highsmith, Andrew R. "Beyond Corporate Abandonment: General Motors and
    the Politics of Metropolitan Capitalism in Flint, Michigan." *Journal of Urban
    History* 40, no. 1 (2014): 35. Accessed January 1, 2016. EBSCO.

50. Goodman, Amy. "What Did GM & the Governor Know? GM Stopped Using
    Flint Water Over a Year Before Emergency Declared." *Democracy Now!* February
    17, 2016. Accessed May 1, 2016. http://www.democracynow.org/2016/2/17/
    what_did_gm_the_governor_know.

51. Fogel, Helen. "GM To Close 11 Plants, Idling 29,000." *Philly.com*. Novem-
    ber 7, 1986. Accessed May 1, 2016. http://articles.philly.com/1986-11-07/
    news/26093327_1_gm-truck-chevrolet-pontiac-canada-plants.

52. Covert, Bryce. "How Racism And Anti-Tax Fervor Laid The Groundwork For
    Flint's Water Crisis." *Think Progress*. February 3, 2016. Accessed May 1, 2016.
    http://thinkprogress.org/economy/2016/02/03/3745246/flint-water-cri
    sis-history/.

53. Fine, Sidney. "Michigan and Housing Discrimination, 1949-1968." *Michigan Historical Review* 23, no. 2 (Fall 1997): 100. Accessed May 1, 2016. https://www.law.msu.edu/clinics/rhc/MI_Housing_Disc.pdf.

54. Skidmore, Mark, and Eric Scorsone. "Causes and Consequences of Fiscal Stress in Michigan Cities." *Regional Science and Urban Economics* 41 (2011): 360. Accessed January 1, 2016. doi:10.1016/0166-0462(75)90011-3.

55. Faust, Kasey M., Dulcy M. Abraham, and Shawn P. McElmurry. "Water and Wastewater Infrastructure Management in Shrinking Cities." *Public Works Management & Policy*, 2015, 1-29. Accessed January 1, 2016. EBSCO.

56. State of Michigan. Emergency Manager Factsheet. Accessed February 15, 2016. https://www.michigan.gov/documents/snyder/EMF_Fact_Sheet2_347889_7.pdf.

57. Lorie, Julia. "What Flint's Dirty Water and Detroit's Angry Teachers Have in Common." *Mother Jones.* January 28, 2016. Accessed February 03, 2016. http://www.motherjones.com/politics/2016/01/emergency-managers-michigan-flint-detroit.

58. Ibid.

59. Ibid.

60. Kozacek, Codi. "Michigan DEQ's Responsibility to Ensure Public Safety Collapsed in Flint." RSS. January 25, 2016. Accessed February 03, 2016. http://www.resilience.org/stories/2016-01-25/michigan-deq-s-responsibility-to-ensure-public-safety-collapsed-in-flint.

61. "How Michigan's Bureaucrats Created the Flint Water Crisis." *Fortune.* Accessed April 03, 2016. http://fortune.com/flint-water-crisis/.

62. Fonger, Ron. "Schuette ups the ante in Flint water crisis with new manslaughter charges." MLive. Accessed on August 1, 2017. http://www.mlive.com/news/flint/index.ssf/2017/06/schuette_ups_the_ante_in_flint.html

63. World Health Organization. "Exposure to Lead: A Major Public Health Concern." Preventing Disease Through Healthy Environments. 2010. Accessed April 27, 2016. http://www.who.int/ipcs/features/lead..pdf?ua=1.

64. Egan, Paul. "Flint Water Mystery: How Was Decision Made?" *Detroit Free Press.* November 22, 2015. Accessed December 10, 2015. http://www.freep.com/story/news/politics/2015/11/21/snyders-top-aide-talked-flint-water-supply-alternatives/76037130/.

65. World Health Organization. "Exposure to Lead: A Major Public Health Concern." Preventing Disease Through Health Environments. 2010. Accessed April

27, 2016. http://www.who.int/ipcs/features/lead..pdf?ua=1.http://www. who.int/ipcs/features/lead..pdf?ua=1.

66. IPCS. (1995). *Inorganic lead.* Geneva, World Health Organization, International Programme on Chemical Safety (Environmental Health Criteria 165; http://www.inchem.org/documents/ehc/ehc/ehc165.htm).

67. Mcnutt, Maria. "Economics of Public Safety." *Science* 351, no. 6274 (February 12, 2016): 641. Accessed January 1, 2016. doi:10.1126/science.aaf4014.

68. EPA. Drinking Water Infrastructure Needs Assessment and Survey: Fifth Report to Congress. 2011. Accessed April 12, 2016. https://www.epa.gov/sites/production/files/2015-07/documents/epa816r13006.pdf.

69. Weesjes, Elke. "Flint Crisis Hasn't Steeled the Nation Against the Health Risks of Lead." *Natural Hazards Observer.* March 2016.

70. ASCE. Report Card for America's Infrastructure. 2013. Accessed April 12, 2016. http://www.infrastructurereportcard.org/; EPA. Drinking Water Infrastructure Needs Assessment and Survey: Fifth Report to Congress. 2011. Accessed April 12, 2016. https://www.epa.gov/sites/production/files/2015-07/documents/epa816r13006.pdf.

71. EPA. Summary of the Safe Drinking Water Act. October 8, 2015. Accessed April 12, 2016. https://www.epa.gov/laws-regulations/summary-safe-drinking-water-act; ASCE. Report Card for America's Infrastructure. 2013. Accessed April 12, 2016. http://www.infrastructurereportcard.org/; EPA. Drinking Water Infrastructure Needs Assessment and Survey: Fifth Report to Congress. 2011. Accessed April 12, 2016. https://www.epa.gov/sites/production/files/2015-07/documents/epa816r13006.pdf.

72. 100 Resilient Cities. Accessed March 1, 2016. http://www.100resilientcities.org/#/-_/.

Sources for Table

Congress. "H.R. 4479 - Families of Flint Act." All Actions: H.R.4479—114th Congress (2015-2016). February 4, 2016. Accessed April 27, 2016. https://www.congress.gov/bill/114th-congress/house-bill/4479/all-actions?overview=closed.

Covert, Bryce. "How Racism And Anti-Tax Fervor Laid The Groundwork For Flint's Water Crisis." *Think Progress.* February 3, 2016. Accessed May 1, 2016. http://thinkprogress.org/economy/2016/02/03/3745246/flint-water-crisis-history/.

Egan, Paul. "Flint Water Mystery: How Was Decision Made?" *Detroit Free Press.* November 22, 2015. Accessed December 10, 2015. http://www.freep.com/story/

news/politics/2015/11/21/snyders-top-aide-talked-flint-water-supply-alterna
tives/76037130/.

Koerner, Claudia. "EPA Official Resigns Over Flint, Michigan, Water Crisis." *Buzz-
feed News*, January 21, 2016. Accessed April 27, 2016. https://www.buzzfeed.com/
claudiakoerner/epa-official-resigns-over-flint-michigan-water-crisis?utm_term=
.qsN2WE05N#.elKEa5Kql.

Lead in Flint, Michigan's Drinking Water: Federal Regulatory Role United States
Congressional Research Service, Specialist in Environmental Policy, March 2, 2016,
CRS.

CHAPTER 5

THE ENVIRONMENTAL PRICE OF INTERGOVERNMENTAL FAILURE IN FLINT

Megan M. DeMasters

Introduction

In the United States, because power and authority to pass and implement policy is shared between various levels of government, understanding the working relations between levels of government is of the utmost importance. In particular, environmental laws require high levels of trust, communication, and cooperation between said levels of government to ensure that they are implemented effectively. More specifically, laws related to drinking water quality such as the Safe Drinking Water Act (SDWA) highlight both the complexities of implementing federal laws at the state level, and questions regarding which level of government should be held accountable when it fails to provide safe drinking water and instead provides water that is toxic to its citizens.

The recent water crisis in Flint, Michigan, illustrates the severe risk contaminated drinking water poses to public health and safety and has been the subject of much debate over which level of government should be held responsible. Looking through the lens of intergovernmental relations, the purpose of this chapter is to provide a greater understanding of the Flint water crisis and the breakdown in the implementation of the Safe Drinking Water Act. In doing so, this chapter utilizes concepts from Scheberle's (2004) implementation model, which argues that federal-state working relations affect the ability of states to adequately implement and enforce federal policy related to environmental laws, including drinking water quality.[1] Specifically, through analysis of secondary documentation, this chapter illustrates that the Flint water crisis reflects a working relationship between levels of government that is described as "contentious and coming apart," thus resulting in the failure of government at all levels.

This chapter proceeds by providing a brief primer on the SDWA, focusing on elements of the Act directly relating to Flint. Next, the relevant implementation literature will be reviewed, specifically focusing on literature and studies pertaining to intergovernmental implementation. Third, this chapter will review case information by level of government, highlighting the role each level played in the Flint water crisis. After a brief overview of the Flint crisis, elements from Scheberle's implementation model will be used to analyze the breakdown in intergovernmental working relations with respect to enforcing federal drinking water standards. This chapter will conclude with some final thoughts for practitioners and academics alike.

Brief Primer to the Safe Drinking Water Act

Due to many environmental concerns during the 1970s, including concerns over the quality of drinking water across the United States, in 1974, Congress passed the Safe Drinking Water Act (SDWA). The SDWA authorizes the Environmental Protection Agency (EPA) to establish national standards for potable drinking water and is designed to protect public health from both natural and anthropogenic threats to water quality.[2] To ensure water quality standards, the EPA requires public water systems to meet several technological and water treatment requirements. For example, the 1991 Lead and Copper Rule (LCR) aims to protect the health of the public by reducing the amount of lead and copper in drinking water sources.[3] To ensure public water systems comply with this rule, the EPA has published rigorous water testing and sampling guidelines. These guidelines include: identifying when water systems have copper or lead levels higher than what the LCR allows, informing the public when water systems are at dangerous levels, providing education on what the potential health risks are associated with the pollutants, and working in a timely manner to replace water lines if necessary.[4] Of particular importance, a section of the LCR requires public water systems to implement corrosion control treatment (CCT) to ensure lead and copper levels in water sources are minimized.[5]

The SDWA and subsequent rules to ensure water quality such as the LCR are considered partial-preemption programs, which means states must demonstrate that they can both meet and enforce standards set by the federal government to be granted primary enforcement authority.[6] This requires state administrators implementing the SDWA to effectively oversee and manage public water systems responsible for testing and treating drinking water. Additionally, state drinking water programs are also required by the SDWA to ensure that public water systems that do not meet drinking water standards notify residents they serve, and that they take remedial actions when systems are out of compliance with drinking water standards.[7] Because the SDWA is a partial preemption program that promotes intergovernmental utilization, it gives authority to the EPA to enforce the Act when states are not meeting these requirements. Specifically, section 1414 of the SDWA provides authority to the EPA to act when they find a public water system out of compliance. The process of enforcement has several components; first, the EPA notifies the state and public water system of the violation. Second, if the state still has not taken appropriate measures, the EPA issues an order to comply. Finally, section 1431 of the SDWA provides the EPA authority to act when a known threat to safe drinking water "may present an imminent and substantial endangerment to the health of persons, and that appropriate state and local authorities have not acted to protect the health of such persons, the EPA administrator may take such actions as he or she deem necessary to protect the health of such persons."[8] In sum, the nature of the SDWA exemplifies intergovernmental implementation and requires coordination among levels of government. The literature provides a rich context for understanding factors that affect intergovernmental implementation and intergovernmental execution of policy.

A Brief Introduction to Implementation

Implementation studies are key to public administration and policy because they highlight the challenges that street-level implementers face when laws, regulations, and policies are executed. Implementation is defined broadly as the step between government institutions and actors taken to determine that they need to address a problem, and the various factors affecting the execution of policy.[9] Beginning with the first series of implementation studies during the 1970s, the primary aim was to discover what factors contributed to policy failure, or the ineffective execution of public policy.[10] The focus of these studies was top-down, meaning scholars began with the assumption that implementation requires clear hierarchical controls, and administrators responsible for executing policy should have a clear understanding of the policy, as well as the tools necessary to implement various policies effectively. Through case-study analysis of federal policies that are put into use by states, early scholars of implementation found that implementation failure was often the result of the federal government setting unrealistic or unattainable goals. Moreover, scholars of the time asserted there was a need for a more systematic understanding of implementation and factors contributing to its failure.[11] Examples of early implementation studies highlighting the disconnect between what the federal government wants done and how implementation occurred include Derthick's 1972[12] study examining application of federal programs addressing social and economic issues associated with urban sprawl, as well as Pressman and Wildavsky's work, which finds that joint action among different actors and levels of government is a major obstacle to implementation because of coordination issues.[13]

While these early studies serve as the launching point for all other implementation studies, they are viewed as incomplete because they do not consider the administrators responsible for the execution of programs, including the day-to-day activities and challenges they face. It has been argued that early implementation studies also fail to account for how local actors and socioeconomic environments effect implementation. To account for these factors, scholars attempted a new approach to the study of implementation often categorized as the "bottom-up" approach to implementation studies.

Bottom-up approaches to implementation assert that these studies should begin with street-level bureaucrats, focusing on understanding the relationships and interactions among street-level implementing staff, their environment, and other groups that they interact with. Beginning with an examination of street-level bureaucrats and their day-to-day activities, scholars using this approach find that policy change is inevitable due to street level administrators need to adapt to their political and environmental situations.[14]

The main criticism of the bottom-up approach to implementation is the emphasis it places on street-level administrators without adequately recognizing how laws, norms within agencies and resources (or lack thereof) affect implementation actions.[15] Recognizing the limitations of both the top-down and bottom-up approaches to implementation, scholars moved towards synthesizing the two approaches to provide a more comprehensive understanding of the multitude of factors that affect implementation. Specifically, in examining implementation of federal laws and regulations at the state level, several scholars have argued that intergovernmental working relationships, coupled with contextual factors and lack of financial or other incentives (among other factors) for states to effectively implement federal laws, contribute to the complexity of implementation of federal policies at the state level.[16]

78

In her book *Federalism and Environmental Policy*, Scheberle offers a comprehensive model of implementation, incorporating factors from both top-down and bottom-up implementation approaches in intergovernmental contexts. Strengths of Scheberle's approach to studying implementation include recognition that implementation becomes much more complex when multiple levels of government are involved. Through the incorporation of both extrinsic (factors outside of an implementing agencies' control) and intrinsic factors (implementing agencies have some control over) into her model, Scheberle acknowledges that unique contextual and intergovernmental settings affect implementation outcomes.

Table 1. Extrinsic and Intrinsic Factors Relating to Intergovernmental Implementation (Adapted from Scheberle 2004, 44)

Extrinsic Factors	*Intrinsic Factors*
Political leadership and support	Intergovernmental Working Relations
Role orientation of oversight agency personnel	Role orientation of agency personnel
Nature of the problem	Agency Capacity
Available resources	Agency Culture
Statutory and Regulatory language including the extent of change in that language	Relationship to the group affected by laws or regulations
Judicial interpretations	Implementation energizer
Demands for change	Resistance to change
Linkages to other laws and programs	

Not only does Scheberle develop a model which identifies various factors affecting implementation, but she also creates a typology of working relationships between the federal government and states acting as the primary implementer of federal environmental laws. Scheberle argues that successful implementation of federal regulations at the state level requires both high levels of trust between state and federal actors, and high levels of involvement of federal oversight personnel with state-implementing agencies. Based on these characteristics, the typology outlines four possible types of working relationships between the federal government and states. First, Scheberle argues that relationships that have both high trust and high involvement represent a relationship of "pulling together," and is the type of relationship that both federal and state level implementers should strive for. The relationship can be characterized as symbiotic, in which "involvement is based on a shared commitment to the policy objectives and a common recognition of the nature of the public problem to be solved." The second type of relationship is "cooperative but not autonomous," having high trust but low levels of involvement. Third is "coming apart with avoidance," which has low trust and low involvement; and finally, relationships characterized by low trust and high levels of federal involvement are defined as "coming apart and contentious."

High trust		
	Cooperative but autonomous	Pulling together and synergistic
Low Trust		
	Coming apart with avoidance	Coming apart and contentious
	Low Involvement	High Involvement

Figure 1. Typology of Federal-State Working Relationships
(Adapted from Scheberle 2004; 22)

In sum, Scheberle's approach to intergovernmental implementation is particularly useful when analyzing the failure of government in the Flint case because the model specifically examines how implementation of federal environmental laws unfold across states. Each of the major relevant extrinsic and intrinsic factors will be discussed in the context of Flint and how they contributed to breakdown of intergovernmental implementation of federal drinking water laws and regulations.

The Role of Levels of Government in Relation to the Flint Water Crisis

The Flint water crisis has been described by many as one of the most egregious failures of government to protect public health, and the greatest environmental justice issue of our time.[17] Administrators at every level of government were quick to point fingers, arguing that administrators at other levels of government should have done more to prevent the crisis. This was a failure of all levels of government to implement and execute federal drinking water standards. Moreover, this failure has far-reaching consequences for implementers at all levels of government and society.

To summarize, the city of Flint was on the verge of bankruptcy. The city council and state-appointed emergency manager agreed that by switching their water source from the Detroit Water and Sewage Department (DWSD), the city could save money. It was decided that Flint would join the Karegnondi Water Authority (KWA), a newly established water authority which was in the process of building a pipeline. While the switch was projected to save the region $200 million dollars over 25 years,[18] the city still needed an interim water source. Administrators decided that while waiting for the KWA to become operational, the city would receive water from the Flint River and the Flint Water Treatment plant, would be re-opened, as it had been closed for many years. However, in this effort to save money, state administrators failed to ensure the water was safe for human consumption. More specifically, administrators failed to put corrosion control measures in place, resulting in drinking water contamination from rust, iron and lead from the pipes.[19]

Almost immediately after water was delivered from the Flint water treatment plant, residents began complaining about the smell, color, and taste of their drinking water. Despite repeatedly being told by local and state administrators the water was safe to drink, residents began getting sick, many of which will continue to suffer long term effects of drinking the water. Because the responsibility to ensure safe drinking water is shared between levels of government, beginning with the Environmental Protection Agency (EPA), the following section provides a brief and general overview of the role that federal, state, and local governments play in securing safe and healthy drinking water. More importantly, this section will explore how they failed to ensure safe water in Flint, Michigan.

Environmental Protection Agency

The EPA has ten regional offices across the country, each of which are responsible for working with states in their regions to support and coordinate efforts for environmental protection. EPA Region Five is responsible for working with Michigan. In June 2015, Miguel Del Toral, a drinking water regulations manager for the region, was contacted by residents complaining about the taste, smell and looks of their drinking water. Miguel Del Toral responded to the complaint and upon testing the water, found that toxin levels related to lead and copper were too high. Del Toral filed a report indicating that there were elevated levels of lead in residential water supplies and recommended immediate action.[20] Despite Del Toral's recommendation and supporting data indicating toxic lead levels, the EPA failed to act at that time. Moreover, the report, once made public by the EPA, left out crucial details about the levels of toxins in the water, and the EPA continued to allow Michigan's Department of Environmental Quality take the lead on water quality.

The EPA maintains that they were working "behind the scenes" with the state of Michigan to remedy the water quality issues, while still allowing residents of Flint to drink the water. It was not until the water crisis was made public that the EPA took enforcement action. The EPA issued an emergency order in January of 2016 expanding federal oversight due to "serious and ongoing concern with the safety of Flint's drinking water system and continuing delay and lack of transparency."[21]

While the EPA ultimately took over administering and enforcing the SDWA, it has been argued that the EPA's response was "too little, too late." and that the EPA should have acted sooner to enforce the SDWA. In sum, while the EPA is not the primary permitting authority for most states, due to partial preemption, they maintain legal authority to supersede state and local authorities when threats to drinking water are imminent. Moreover, because the EPA was contacted by residents of Flint concerning water quality, they had an obligation to act.

Michigan Department of Environmental Quality

In the final report written by the Flint Water Advisory Task Force, responsibility for the contaminated water in Flint was assigned to the Michigan Department of Environmental Quality (MDEQ).[22] The task force asserts that the MDEQ is primarily responsible for the crisis because the state of Michigan and the MDEQ by extension had achieved primacy to implement the SDWA. In other words, the MDEQ was the primary agency responsible for ensuring standards for safe drinking water were met. More specifically, the task force highlights the role of the Office of Drinking Water and Municipal Assistance's (ODWMA) within the MDEQ, whose primary function is "regulatory oversight of the approximately 1,425 community public water supplies in Michigan."[23]

When determining where water should come from to supply the city of Flint, administrators from the MDEQ discussed the health risks associated with using water from the Flint River and because of these concerns, agreed that the Flint River should not be considered a permanent water source. However, despite the known health risks, and the fact that the Flint Water Treatment Plant had not been operating for many years, administrators agreed that with some improvements water from the Flint River could be used as a temporary source while Flint transitioned from the DWSD to the KWA.[24] While the MDEQ did set up initial water testing periods during the first six months the Flint Water Treatment Plant was operational, it was determined that corrosion control measures to protect the water from lead and copper pipe corrosion was not immediately necessary. Rather, the MDEQ decided they would test the water again and determine the need for corrosion control technology after the plant had been operational for six months. In December of 2014, six months after residents had begun drinking water from the Flint River, the MDEQ found that the water quality was out of compliance with the SDWA Disinfection and Byproduct rule. Further testing also indicated that levels of lead and copper were high. This indicates that the plant should not have been exempted from corrosion standards. Despite this, the MDEQ failed to direct operators of the Flint Water Treatment Plant to implement corrosion control standards. Additionally, after the EPA got involved, it was discovered that staff from the MDEQ were not testing water for pollutants according to federal standards, minimizing what looked like the risk for contaminated water.

In sum, several e-mails, and other documentation highlight that the MDEQ had knowledge that the water from the Flint River was not safe to drink, but chose to deliver the water despite knowing the health risks. Moreover, the MDEQ did not follow appropriate protocols to ensure the water was safe, resulting in health, ecological, and other effects.[25]

The City of Flint

Under the SDWA, operators of public water systems are responsible for ensuring their systems comply with SDWA standards. In this case, the City of Flint was responsible for maintaining compliance with the SDWA because Flint owns the public water system that was utilized to supply water from the Flint River to residents. Crucial components for the Flint Water Treatment Plant (WTP) include "ensuring proper design, construction and operations and maintenance, so that contaminants in tap water do not exceed the standards established by law."[26] To remain in compliance, the city is "required to employ properly certified water operators that are trained and experienced to operate the treatment and distribution system."[27] As noted earlier, because Flint came under the authority of a state appointed emergency manager, city officials had little authority when making these decisions. However, they remain culpable in several ways. First, the Public Works department was the government agency in Flint at the frontline of monitoring water quality in the system. Next, the city was responsible for ensuring that the WTP was upgraded and tested to ensure that it could operate effectively, ensuring that staff members were properly trained, including being familiar with treatment processes, and maintaining the technology to ensure drinking water was safe. In sum, Flint does have some responsibility in the water crisis because they operated the public water system in their role as public water system operators. However, the employees there lacked experience in water quality treatment to adequately ensure the water met the standards of the SDWA. Moreover, like many other communities in Michigan, Flint relied heavily on support from the MDEQ staff to guide them on how best to meet standards. Therefore, lack of support from the MDEQ coupled with limited experience on the part of city staff resulted in failure to meet water quality standards.

It is recognized that there may be other agencies that have some culpability with the Flint crisis. However, for this chapter, and in relation to the implementation and enforcement of the SDWA, those described here are the most relevant. It is also recognized that there are many details that have been left out when discussing the role of these levels of government; again, the purpose here is to focus on general background to serve in explaining the crisis in the context of intergovernmental implementation failure.

Explaining the Flint Water Crisis in the Context of Intergovernmental Implementation

While many factors may explain implementation failure in Flint, utilizing Scheberle's implementation model, only the intrinsic and extrinsic factors that best explain the implementation failure will be discussed. Extrinsic factors include the availability of resources, statutory and regulatory language, and the role of the EPA as the oversight agency. Intrinsic factors examined are agency capacity and intergovernmental working relations.

Extrinsic Factors

Availability of Resources. Availability of resources is a factor that continues to challenge implementers of federal drinking water standards because often, implementers and public water systems required to test and maintain certain technology to ensure safe drinking water do not have the financial resources to do so. Lack of financial resources affects state implementation in several ways, including the cost of keeping small water systems in compliance, costs of building new infrastructure, and the cost of replacing old or aging infrastructure.[28] In a report released by ASDWA in conjunction with the EPA, it was estimated that total costs needed to meet minimum standards of the Act were $625 million and $785 million. However, state reported funding for fiscal year 2013 was $385 million for base programs and $440 million for comprehensive programs, representing a funding gap of $240 million for base programs and $308 million for comprehensive programs.[29] In addition to this, contracts cities have with public water suppliers are, in large part, a financial decision. This was the case with the water supply in Flint. For the city of Flint, the exorbitant cost of receiving drinking water from the DWSD highlights how socioeconomics affects access to safe, clean water.[30] Flint could not afford to pay the high rates for water, which is why they switched sources in the first place. This highlights a bigger issue— availability (or inability of resources) affects equitable distribution of safe drinking water. Flint having a largely poor and minority community has led to this crisis being characterized by Paul Mohai, an environmental justice scholar, as the "one of the biggest environmental justice disasters I know."[31]

Statutory and Regulatory Language. How a law or regulation is written can greatly affect implementation of that law, mainly because regulatory language is often vague, without clear jurisdictional guidelines. The interpretation of federal drinking water regulations caused actors at all levels of government to point fingers, placing blame on the other, without taking full responsibility for their own actions. The response of both the State of Michigan and the EPA to the Flint crisis is illustrative of this. For example, despite the initial complaint of concern with water quality being received by the EPA, they failed to act in a timely manner. EPA Region Five employee Susan Headman maintains, however, that based on how federal regulations are written, the EPA did nothing wrong, arguing that the EPA had "limited enforcement actions."[32] Moreover, Hedman testified during the Congressional hearing on Flint, Michigan, that she worked within the legal framework by asking state and local government to act. While Hedman maintains that the EPA acted within the scope of federal drinking water regulations because the SDWA is a partial preemption program, when it was evident that the MDEQ was not complying with federal drinking water standards, the EPA had both the authority and obligation to act. Despite the EPA's authority to act, the ambiguous language of the SDWA and failure to specify when the EPA should act was viewed as an underlying issue in the Flint water crisis.

To ensure that a catastrophe like Flint does not occur again, Congress has passed several amendments to the SDWA. These amendments outline the roles and duties of the EPA when a state or public water system is not complying with federal drinking water standards. In addition to these amendments, the House of Representatives has since passed a bill clearly outlining roles and duties of the EPA when a system is found to be out of compliance to ensure that a catastrophe like Flint does not happen again.

Role of the Oversight Agency. Because the SDWA and the lead and copper rule under the SDWA are considered partial preemption programs, it has generally been agreed that the EPA had a responsibility to act earlier in the case of Flint to enforce drinking water standards set forth in the SDWA. This lends credence to the fact that most people felt that the EPA should be taking more enforcement actions to do their job.[33] Additionally, Del Toral, the EPA employee who first tested the water, wrote "at every stage of this process, it seems that we spend more time trying to maintain state/local relationships than we do trying to protect children."[34] This suggests the view of the EPA's role was as an equal team member, rather than recognizing their superior role in the SDWA.

Intrinsic Factors

Agency Capacity. At both the state and local levels, agencies did not have the technical expertise, personnel, or funds available to adequately do their jobs. First, the MDEQ, where most of the blame has fallen has since publicly acknowledged that they applied the wrong standards when testing the water.[35] Next, city employees responsible for operating the public water system were not adequately trained in how to operate the Flint water treatment plant. This resulted in failure to apply the appropriate water treatment techniques. Even though city employees did not apply the appropriate techniques, most of the blame still falls on the MDEQ, specifically the ODW-MA branch, because it is part of the agency's responsibility to ensure that city-level employees are trained properly. Recently, administrators from the MDEQ have taken responsibility, admitting that they were not adequately prepared when the water supply source was switched to the Flint River.[36] In sum, both the city of Flint and the MDEQ lacked agency capacity to adequately comply with safe drinking water standards.

Relationship to Group Affected by Laws or Regulations. In the case of Flint, the group that was most directly affected by the laws and regulations are the people who were the most affected by failure to comply with water quality regulations—residents of Flint. The regulatory agencies responsible for complying with drinking water standards did not maintain a trustful relationship with their residents. After the switch of the water supply to the Flint River, MDEQ staff continued to assure residents that the water was safe, allowing them to continue using it for an extended period of time. Next, although the water was found to be unsafe, the EPA did not act in a timely manner. The EPA's unwillingness to take enforcement action on the MDEQ resulted in residents drinking contaminated water for a longer period, suggesting that both EPA staff and MDEQ staff held little regard for the health and welfare of Flint residents whom they have a responsibility under the law to protect.[37]

Intergovernmental Working Relations. In Scheberle's assessment of the SDWA (2004), she asserts that intergovernmental relations pose the greatest challenge to successful implementation of the SDWA. Scheberle asserts that working relations between federal and state government are characterized as contentious and falling apart. One of the characteristics of working relations that are considered contentious and falling apart is that "communication flows freely but does not often produce satisfying results."[38] The pressure put on the MDEQ and failure of the EPA to act, when it was made clear the MDEQ was not taking the necessary steps to resolve water quality issues, support the characterization of the working relationship as contentious and falling apart. Further support for this characterization includes the decision by region administrators to alter Del Toral's original report to remove information that there were high levels of pollutants, lead, and copper in Flint's water supply. In addition, e-mail correspondence between the EPA and the MDEQ reveal that the EPA, to fix relations, worked "behind the scenes" to put pressure on the MDEQ to act, rather than take punitive action against them. This suggests the EPA prioritized maintaining their working relationship with the MDEQ over the public health and safety concerns of the Flint community. This finding is further supported by Del Toral's testimony to Congress that the EPA prioritized agency relations above public health and safety of Flint residents.[39]

Conclusion

The purpose of this chapter was to illustrate the failure of government at all levels to implement the SDWA, resulting in severe health and environmental problems for Flint. Using an adapted version of Scheberle's intergovernmental implementation model, there are several factors discussed that affected intergovernmental implementation and the failure of government to protect the health of Flint residents. First was the availability of resources. The lack of resources available to replace aging water supply infrastructure is a problem that plagues many public water systems, including Flint's. Second was the vagueness of the statutory language in the SDWA, specifically related to which level of government is ultimately responsible for ensuring the law is being implemented. Third was the proper role of the oversight agency—the regional EPA office. The EPA in this case failed to meet their obligation to ensure the MDEQ was properly implementing the lead and copper rules of the SDWA. The fourth factor discussed was agency capacity—lack of funds, personnel, and training of personnel at the Flint water treatment facility also contributed to the failure of government to respond quickly. Fifth was the relationship between groups targeted by a law or regulation. This chapter showed that the EPA and MDEQ acted in a manner that showed little regard for the residents of Flint, whom they were responsible to for supplying safe drinking water. Finally, this chapter showed that the working relations between the EPA and MDEQ can be characterized as contentious and falling apart. This is based upon evidence suggesting the agencies were in communication, yet did not work together to remedy the water quality issues in Flint. Overall, these factors highlight the failure of government at all levels to respond to the Flint water crisis. The EPA failed to exercise authority to enforce compliance when they were made aware of prohibitive issues. The MDEQ did not require corrosion control measures and failed to adequately prepare the Flint WTP to test water supplies. Finally, while they are the least culpable, the city of Flint failed to ensure their water system was up to code.

Moreover, the failure of government resulted in four primary costs. These costs are first, the cost to the health of the public. Residents of Flint will be suffering from many health-related issues for years to come. Second are the large economic costs. The cost to residents to fix the infrastructure and costs associated with health issues will continue to impact Flint. Third is the loss of trust between citizens and government. Government has an obligation to protect citizens from harm; in this case, failure to act will continue to result in loss of trust. The final cost is the loss of trust among implementers across all levels of government. The costs of intergovernmental failure in this case suggest that future federal, state, and local government should consider costs of inaction, and ensure that they are working cooperatively to implement laws and regulations that will continue to protect citizens.

Notes

1. Scheberle, Denise. 2004. *Federalism and Environmental Policy: Trust and The Politics of Implementation*. Fourth Edition, Georgetown University Press.

2. Environmental Protection Agency. 2012. "Safe Drinking Water Act."

3. Environmental Protection Agency. 2016. "Lead and Copper Rule."

4. Davis, Matthew M., Chris Kolb, Lawrence Reynolds, Eric Rothstein, & Ken Sikkema. "Flint Water Advisory Task Force Final Report." 2016. Office of Governor Rick Snyder, State of Michigan.

5. Environmental Protection Agency. 2008. "Lead and Copper Rule: Quick Reference Guide."

6. Vig, Norman, & Kraft, Michael E. 2009. *Environmental Politics & Policy*, 7th ed. Eds. Norman Vig and Michael E. Kraft. Washington, DC: CQ Press.

7. Environmental Protection Agency. 2004. "Protecting Drinking Water Sources"; Environmental Protection Agency. 2004a. "Drinking Water Treatment."

8. *Safe Drinking Water Act of 1974*. Public Law 93-533. 42 USC. 300j-25.

9. O'Toole, Laurence J., Jr. 2000. "Research on Policy Implementation: Assessment and Prospects." *Journal of Public Administration Research and Theory* 20: 263-88.

10. Hood, C. (1976). *The limits of administration*. London; Toronto: Wiley.

11. Smith, K. B., & Larimer, C. W. 2013. *The Public Policy Theory Primer*. Boulder, CO: Westview Press; Chang Yu-Min. 1999. *Factors contributing to the effectiveness of implementing a national policy at the local level: A case study of community-specific regulation of municipal water pollution control*. Proquest Dissertation and Theses Global.

12. Derthick, Martha. 1972. *New Towns In-Town*. Urban Institute Press Washington D.C.

13. Pressman, L. Jeffrey, & Wildavsky, Aaron. 1973. *Implementation*. University of California Press, Berkeley.

14. Majone, G., & Wildavsky, A. (1984). Implementation as evolution: Exorcising the ghost in the implementation machine. *Russell Sage Discussion Papers*, (2).

15. Sabatier, P. A. 1986. Top-down and bottom-up approaches to implementation research: a critical analysis and suggested synthesis. *Journal of Public Policy*, 6 (1), 21-48.

16. Pressman, L. Jeffrey, & Wildavsky, Aaron. 1973. *Implementation*. University of California Press, Berkeley; Derthick, Martha. 1972. *New Towns In-Town*. Urban Institute Press Washington D.C.

17. Bernstein, Lenny, & Dennis Brady. "Flint's water crisis reveals government failures at every level." *Washington Post*, January 24, 2016.

18. Shapiro, Ari. "Flint residents' broken faith: "The people we trusted failed us."" NPR, February 10, 2016.

19. Bernstein & Brady, 2016.

20. Spangler, Todd. "Emails shed light on EPA's role in Flint water crisis." *Detroit Free Press*, March 5, 2016.

21. Goodnough, Abby. "House Panel Denounces E.P.A. Actions in Flint Crisis." March 15, 2016.

22. Davis, et al. 2016.

23. Ibid.

24. Ibid.

25. Ibid.; Spangler, Todd. 2016.

26. Davis, et al. 2016.

27. Ibid.

28. Association of State Drinking Water Administrators. 2013. "Insufficient Resources for State Drinking Water Programs Threaten Public Health: An Analysis of State Drinking Water Programs' Resources and Needs."

29. Ibid.

30. Davis, et al. 2016.

31. Bernstein & Brady, 2016.

32. Goodnough, 2016.

33. Lynch, Jim. "Michigan DEQ vows changes in Flint water crisis." October 19, 2015; Sanburn, J. (2016). "Flint Water Crisis May Cost the City $400 Million in Long-Term Social Costs."

34. Del Toral, 2015, as quoted by Goodnough 2016. "House Panel Denounces E.P.A. Actions in Flint Crisis." March 15, 2016.

35. Lynch. 2015.

36. Ibid.

37. Bernstein & Brady. 2016.

38. Scheberle. 2004.

39. Goodnough. 2016.

CHAPTER 6

INCREASING RESILIENCE TO SLOW-ONSET EVENTS: THE CASE OF FLINT

Christine Pommerening

Introduction

Emergency management is, by necessity, oriented towards concrete and discrete events—as pre-event planning and preparedness, and post-event response and recovery. Slow-onset events like pandemics, poisoning, or pollution, are the "known unknowns" of risk assessment and emergency management. Unlike other disasters or disruptions, slow-onset event incidence or even existence is not easily and immediately observable.[1] Comprehensive discussions of technological disasters and their environmental safety and public health aspects usually refer to rapid-onset industrial disasters, such as Bhopal and Chernobyl.[2] While nuclear contamination, for example, has long been part of disaster planning, it is assumed to be directly tied to a sudden adverse event like a reactor meltdown or a dirty bomb designed to spread radioactive material throughout a specific area.

The difference to slow-onset events is both time and space—slow-onset is harder to discover but potentially preventable, yet unlike most other hazards, distance to the source does not matter here, thus defying typical response operations. Threats, vulnerabilities, and consequences that result from societal, structural, or systemic features are more difficult to include in a typical emergency management framework.

Slow-onset events have more in common with long-term humanitarian crisis management than with domestic incident management. The former is typically the domain of international aid organizations and involves, among other things, providing hunger relief, building refugee camps, and resettling populations. For the latter, the U.S. has developed a comprehensive federal planning base, including the National Infrastructure Protection Plan, the National Incident Management System, and the National Planning Frameworks, all of which establish roles and responsibilities for public agencies first and foremost, but also the private sector and the public at large.[3, 4, 5]

The Flint Water Crisis falls in between these two approaches: it is a long-term, structural problem in an already-distressed community, as well as an infrastructure failure. Thus, any solution needs to address both aspects. The principle and practice of resilience, as societal resilience and as infrastructure resilience, provides such a common framework for a solution. This chapter will examine the crisis as a slow-onset event, assess its specific community and infrastructure characteristics, and outline decision points to deal with similar crises in the future.

Resilience in Systems and Organizations

The problem of effective coordination of disaster preparedness and response under conditions of uncertainty is similar to the problems addressed in organizational analyses of infrastructure systems. In fact, many studies in this discipline use examples from public and private organizations that have to deal with natural or technological hazards, and use those case studies to explain factors influencing risk management and response capabilities. There is a large body of literature in the social sciences, as well as operations research and engineering, on various aspects contributing to (or diminishing) the resilience of systems. In this section, three examples will be discussed that are representative of prominent concepts in the social sciences: first, normal accidents; second, complex adaptive systems; and third, societal safety and risk perception.

Normal Accidents

Studies on the prevention of industrial accidents have traditionally been the domain of safety engineers. The dominant view was not that the engineered systems themselves could be inherently unsafe, but rather that shop floor conditions or operating errors lead to accidents, and that few, if any, negative externalities existed. Triggered by large-scale disruptions such as the accident at the nuclear power plant Three Mile Island in 1979, this view was challenged. In his 1984 book, Charles Perrow used insights from systems design, decision theory, and organizational theory to formulate a theory of failure of systems and, more importantly, recovery from failure.[6]

A system in this sense is an aggregation of components, from units to parts to subsystems. Accordingly, "accidents" are also distinguished in ascending order from incidents to accidents, to component failure accidents to system accidents. While the latter are by far the rarest events, with an empirical frequency of about 1% (based on classifications of Nuclear Regulatory Commission Licensee Event Reports), Perrow argues that these low probability/high consequence events are the most instructive for understanding the multiple points of failure inherent in a system. This includes the equally manifold points of potential pre- or post-event intervention.[7]

Perrow distinguishes systems in degrees of a) interaction, and b) coupling or the amount of "slack, buffer or give between two items. Failures caused by system properties rather than human errors in either design or operation. The eponymous "normal accident theory" thus describes system accidents that "involve the unanticipated interaction of multiple failures."[8]

Complex systems are characterized by spatial proximity, common-mode connections, interconnected subsystems, limited substitutions, feedback loops, multiple and overlapping controls, indirect information, and limited understanding. Examples include nuclear plants, as well as multi-goal agencies, such as the Department of Energy (which has regulatory, research, and commercial functions.) Linear systems are characterized by spatial segregation, dedicated connections, segregated subsystems, easy substitutions, few feedback loops, single-purpose and segregated controls, direct information, and extensive understanding. Examples include dams and rail transportation.

Tight coupling is associated with time-dependent and invariant processes with designed-in buffers only, and little if any slack. Resources cannot be substituted easily or at all. Loose coupling means output delays are possible, and the order of processing can be changed. In such systems, alternative methods and redundant resources are available, and fortuitous buffers and substitutions are possible.

A good example highlighting the differences of "couplings" are different types of power plants. Nuclear plants are tightly-coupled because the sequences are highly invariant, personnel need to be highly trained, and no substitute energy source can be utilized. In contrast, a coal-fired plant can operate with high or low stockpiles of coal, and it can even be switched to other fossil fuels entirely with relatively small adjustments.

The relevance of the coupling concept is that it combines engineering logic with organizational theory, examining the responsiveness of systems to failures and shocks. Understanding a human or technical system's tendencies can help plan the response. There is no *a priori* better or worse type of system, however. Loosely-coupled systems can incorporate shocks and pressures without destabilization because they are somewhat inefficient to begin with. Alternatively, tightly-coupled systems will respond more quickly to changing conditions, but that efficiency may very well turn out to be disastrous.

The important point is that since failures occur in all systems, the means to recovery are critical. Simply put, in tightly-coupled systems, the buffers and redundancies and substitutions must exist already and be part of the design, while in loosely-coupled systems there must be an ability to create solutions on the spot and exploit the system.[9]

Complex Adaptive Systems

Public managers are confronted with increasing risk of potentially catastrophic disruptions in their jurisdictions and need to strengthen the internal capacity of their organizations to prepare for and respond to disasters. In addition, they need to manage interactions with private and nonprofit organizations to protect a community at risk from natural or technological disasters or terrorist attacks. While instruments such as the National Incident Management System and the National Response Framework are supposed to facilitate this coordination, they also reflect the constraints on decision processes under uncertainty, including illustrating the persistent difficulty in achieving coordination among multiple organizations with different responsibilities in different locations.[10]

This type of problem is discussed in complex adaptive system theory. Essentially, it promotes a view of systems as being designed with an ability to adapt to change under conditions of uncertainty—in short, resilience.

In the field of public administration theory, Louise Comfort has examined several cases of disaster planning and recovery.[11] She argues that when public response organizations are under pressure, three elements characterize the types of adaptation to fast-changing conditions. These elements include: technical indicators (e.g., reliability), organizational indicators (e.g., communication and leadership styles), and cultural indicators (e.g., openness to alternative solutions). They vary in degree from non-adaptive to emergent-adaptive to operative-adaptive, and, ideally, auto-adaptive systems.

96

Achieving auto-adaptive systems would require public investment in an information infrastructure that can support the intense demand for communication, information search, exchange, and feedback. This, however. is not only necessary during a disaster, but is also part of day-to-day decision-making. That way, possible risks (threats, vulnerabilities, and consequences) associated with the operation of vital systems can be identified earlier.

Comfort's case study of the inter-organizational disaster response system that evolved following the 1994 Northridge Earthquake showed that striking the balance between preparedness and resilience—order and chaos— is less a matter of an ex-ante planning document or policy decision that stresses the one over the other. Instead, she contends that structuring a process for continuous organizational learning is the primary requirement for maintaining creativity and adaptation when faced with catastrophic events.[12]

Using the notion of complex adaptive systems and their inherent unpredictability, some authors have started to shift focus from managing risk to building resilience.[13] In a study on resilience and communication in unpredictable environments, Patricia Longstaff contends that the rather clinical term "threat" disguises perceptions of danger, uncertainty, and surprise, while "vulnerability" hints at an inherent fragility that is impervious to engineering solutions such as redundancy. She then identifies two main coping strategies for dealing with terrorism, natural disaster, and technology risks: resistance and resilience. Resistance aims at keeping everything safe, such as implied by "fire-resistant" building materials, and is useful when dangers can be anticipated. Prevention, then, is "resistance that keeps bad things from happening." Resilience, on the other hand, is defined as "an individual's, group's, or organization's ability to continue its existence, or to remain more or less stable, in the face of a surprise, either a deprivation of resources or a physical threat."[14]

Societal Safety and Risk Perception

If we assume increasing internal complexity of systems as well as increasing external risks to such systems, then factors such as uncertainty, cognitive limits, and unintended consequences are likely to have an effect beyond their role in a particular organization, technical system, or disaster. In fact, they become important parameters for designing safety and security oriented public policies, per se. This link has been recognized early on by Aaron Wildavsky.[15] He examines how societal approaches to dealing with risk are often ineffective and counterproductive. Generally, he argues, people try to anticipate dangers and then prevent them from causing harm, instead of trying to increase resilience by enhancing the ability to respond to unexpected dangers.[16] He argues that the focus should be shifted from this "passive prevention of harm to a more active search for safety."

He proposes creating a balance of anticipation and resilience as a strategy for reducing risk in uncertain conditions. Anticipation means a careful assessment of vulnerability with prudent action taken to limit obvious danger. This anticipation strategy remains vital to protect against risks whose potential for realization is substantial. Resilience means a flexible response to actual danger, demonstrating an ability to "bounce back" after a damaging event. This resilience strategy is most appropriate for dealing with unexpected events.

A combination of systematic actions to reduce known risks and the capacity to act quickly when faced with unexpected dangers is the most successful resilience strategy. Part of this strategy is to involve the local community by providing information on actual versus perceived risks, and increasing societal coping mechanisms. However, this places a considerable burden on decision makers in that it requires thinking and acting "outside the box" at a time when resources for public information campaigns and community engagement are reduced.

Managing Events and Interventions

Analyzing the characteristics and complex socio-technical systems, both in their routine operations and under extreme conditions and failure, is the first step in formulating a resilience-based risk management plan.

The following schematic and discussion incorporates these characteristics and puts them into a sequential process of empirical needs, choices, hazards, and consequences, as well as potential interventions.[17]

The top level illustrates a sequence with linked empirical events, and the bottom line illustrates potential interventions at different stages. The empirical events may be direct cause-effect relationships, but could also be more general relationships occurring in temporal sequence. The bottom level illustrates potential interventions can be distinguished into monitoring, modifying, and averting, or blocking, of events. The first row in each box is the category of event or intervention, the second row is one example thereof —there are more events that could be listed as well as different interventions, which could then be combined into an event tree. The examples chosen here are explained below.

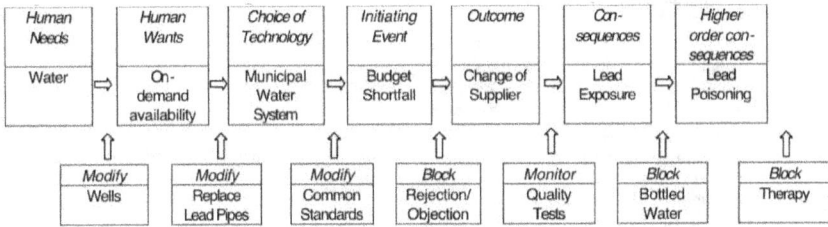

Human Needs	Human Wants	Choice of Technology	Initiating Event	Outcome	Con-sequences	Higher order con-sequences
Water	On-demand availability	Municipal Water System	Budget Shortfall	Change of Supplier	Lead Exposure	Lead Poisoning

Modify	Modify	Modify	Block	Monitor	Block	Block
Wells	Replace Lead Pipes	Common Standards	Rejection/ Objection	Quality Tests	Bottled Water	Therapy

Figure 1. Event Sequence and Intervention Stages

Events

Human Needs and Human Wants. The "Human Needs" and "Human Wants" aspects may seem less of a concern in the context of drinking water supply in Flint and the United States as a developed country, but it is important to recognize that individual and societal needs should determine the priorities for public policy, and, vice versa, not recognizing those basic needs may result in decisions that focus more on technological and administrative expedience. Also, these needs are unfulfilled for millions of people in other parts of the world, and therefore should be considered in risk management as a matter of course.

Choice of Technology. The "Choice of Technology" encompasses a large number of elements, and is, of course, a decisive factor in a technological disaster. One might argue that municipal water system is not actually a choice given its dominance in the provision of water to households in the United States. There are 51,000 Community Water Systems (CWS) that serve residential customers year-round, delivering potable water to over 84 percent of the population (along with smaller and temporary public water systems.) The choice—and complexity—is introduced through the physical, cyber, and human elements that make up a typical water infrastructure system, and which are defined as follows in the Sector-Specific Plan:[18]

99

Water source
This may be groundwater, surface water, or a combination of the two. The vast majority of CWSs serving fewer than ten-thousand people use groundwater as their source. Large CWSs obtain most of their water from surface sources.
Conveyance
To bring water from a remote source to the treatment plant, CWSs may use pipes or open canals; the water may be pumped or gravity-fed.
Raw water storage
Reservoirs or lakes hold water from the source before it is treated; these reservoirs may be in remote or urban areas.
Treatment
A variety of physical and chemical treatments are applied, depending on the contaminants detected in the raw water.
Finished water storage
Treated water is stored before being distributed to customers. In some cases, treated water is stored in large, uncovered reservoirs that may be vulnerable to attack and contamination.
Distribution system
This network of pipes, tanks, pumps, and valves conveys water to customers. The flow is adjusted so that the proper volume and pressure are delivered when and where needed.
Monitoring system
Most monitoring is conducted for conventional regulated and unregulated contaminants. Some utilities have sensors installed at critical points to monitor a range of physical properties, such as water pressure and water quality.
Supervisory Control and Data Acquisition (SCADA) system
Some utilities have electronic networks, often including wireless communication, to link the monitoring system, and controls for the treatment and distribution systems, to a central display in the operations/control room. These systems may also help to automate control of a drinking water utility with monitoring-system readouts serving as inputs for control.
Employees and contractors
Drinking water utilities rely on part-time, full-time, and contract employees to manage and operate their facilities. In larger utilities, this may include chemists, engineers, microbiologists, public relations staff, security personnel, and other specialists. Operators must be appropriately trained and available, typically based on the type, size, and complexity of a utility. Utilities also rely on outside contractors to provide engineering services, laboratory analyses, chemical deliveries, and security services.

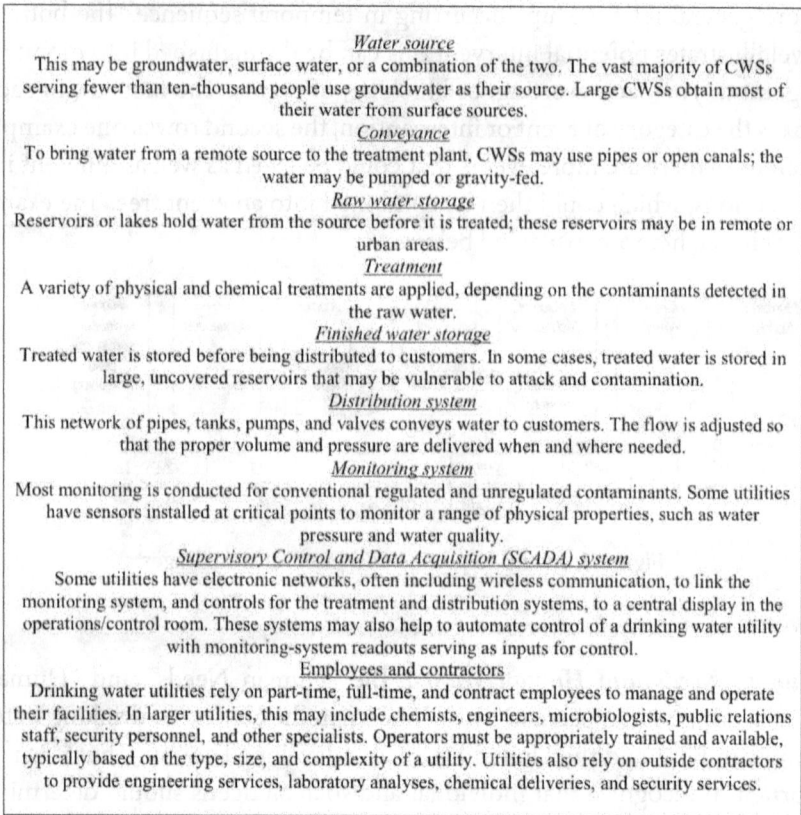

Figure 2. Elements of Community Water Systems

A slow-onset event in a CWS is a sign of a stressed-state system rather than a disrupted or failed system.[19] In fact, the state of operation of an infrastructure is rarely binary ("on or off"), but almost always a continuum from normal operations to stress to disruption to repair and restoration or reconfiguration. At any point in the continuum, the state of operation is a function of the interrelated factors and system conditions. Under certain conditions, an infrastructure can operate at well below the optimal design state (e.g., because one or more units, subsystems, or systems have failed) and still provide what the user perceives as full service, making it more difficult to identify the exact cause and effect of stress.

Initiating Event. The "Initiating Event" in this case is not an external shock, such as a natural disaster or man-made attack, but arguably a financial one that triggered the slow-onset event of lead poisoning. The infrastructure system itself is a vector of disruption, whereas in other disasters the infrastructure is usually the target or loses function as result of cascading failure that started elsewhere.

Here, one might argue that a budget shortfall is hardly a threat on the same level as natural disasters or man-made attacks. Yet as with most disasters or disruptions, it is the coincidence and combination of failures to prevent threats and mitigate vulnerabilities that result in harmful consequences. The budget shortfall is not the only cause, but without it, the decision to switch would have been unlikely, thus making it a key contributor to the sequence of events that followed. Moreover, subsequent decisions by the then newly appointed city emergency manager were also informed by cost-savings considerations (e.g., when a $50,000 investment in corrosion control chemicals was not approved.)[20]

Outcome. The "Outcome," directly tied to the "Initiating Event," is the decision to change water suppliers from the Detroit Water and Sewerage Department (which uses Lake Huron water) to the not-yet operational Karegnondi Water Authority (which will also use Lake Huron water), and switch to its own water treatment plant and Flint River water in the meantime. This system was used only as backup for years, and procedures were not changed, nor were corrosion control chemicals added when it became primary supplier in April 2014.[21]

Consequence. The "Consequence" of the "Outcome" is exposure to lead, due to the higher corrosiveness of Flint River water versus Lake Huron water, and the absence of corrosion control chemicals that could reduce leaching of lead from residential pipes and fixtures. While the exposure started immediately with the switch, the resulting changes were gradual and cumulative, and noticed only over the course of more than a year, making this a slow-onset event.

Higher-Order Consequence. The "Higher-Order Consequence" was lead poisoning observed in vulnerable populations such as children. While multiple concerns were raised and alerts issued starting in late 2014, the first official order was the declaration of a public health emergency by the Genesee County Health Department on October 1, 2015. Subsequent declarations of emergency by the City of Flint, Genesee County, and the State of Michigan in early January 2016 prompted President Obama to declare the first-ever emergency not related to a natural disaster or man-made attack, on January 16, 2016. In that regard, the emergency, once recognized as such, was managed in accordance with established planning frameworks, policy and practice. But the time delay in mobilizing state and federal resources raises fundamental questions of its effectiveness.

Interventions

Modify Source. Switching to a different water source, such as individual wells, is of course impracticable in many cases, and might introduce different contamination risks.[22] The point is that the consideration of alternatives, even as counterfactuals, shows how path-dependent both technological problems and their solutions are.

Modify Delivery. Replacing lead pipes that are common at the residential end of the distribution system is an obvious intervention since their corrosion introduces most of the lead into the tap water. The first step would be to identify those pipes, which property owners can do relatively easily. As a public health concern, the utilities themselves could also provide a web-accessible inventory of such pipes, but many have so far been reluctant to do so, either for lack of data, cost of implementation, or privacy issues.[23]

Modify Policy. Introducing "Common Standards" can refer to a number of interventions, from building codes requiring non-led pipes in new construction or a change in federal lead contamination regulations. Currently, a water system is considered in compliance with the U.S. Environmental Protection Agency's Lead and Copper Rule even if the utility's tests find high levels of lead in up to 10% of customers as determined by occasional samples. This standard might fail to detect "last mile" contamination even if water was being treated properly with chemicals to help control corrosion at the water treatment plant.

Block Decision. At various points after the introduction of a proposal to change suppliers, a rejection or objection by decision-makers on the local, state, and federal levels (from the Flint City Council and Mayor to the Michigan Department of Environmental Quality to the Environmental Protection Agency) could have averted the crisis. It appears that the strongest de facto "objection" came from two counterproposals by the previous supplier, the Detroit Water and Sewerage Authority, to structure a new contract.[24]

Monitor Outcome. The lack of adequate water quality tests is one of the main issues in the ongoing investigation; with adequate testing, the emergency could have been both averted and mitigated. The timing, authority, and recognition of tests by public agencies, private laboratories, and academic researchers, as well as the subsequent potential and actual interventions, has been documented in several oversight hearings before Congress.[25, 26]

Block Consequence. The distribution of bottled water as a way to prevent further lead poisoning is one of the most common means in humanitarian crisis relief and disaster response operations. At this stage, even though the "Initiating Event" is not a typical disaster, there are indeed few alternative interventions. The primacy of preserving human life takes precedent in response efforts, as well as resistant and resilient systems. Although it could be argued that it does not causally follow the prior "Outcome" example of monitoring water quality, the eventual detection of contaminants left bottled water, along with boiling advisories, as the immediate intervention.

Block Higher-Order Consequence. Among the many monitoring, modifying, and blocking options in the emergency response and recovery phase, providing therapy to the affected population and thus mitigating the adverse health effects is arguably the most important one, both immediatly and long-term. It does not alter the events, but, if successful, will allow the affected individuals to physically overcome developmental delays caused by lead poisoning. From a resilience point of view, the interventions dealing with higher consequences are the defining moments for the community at large. Using community resources to self-determine the course of recovery, such as media outreach and political activism, can be a powerful means of both adaptation and change. Among others, LeeAnn Walters, whose persistence eventually led to the discovery and acknowledgment of the lead contamination by authorities, has founded a non-profit community development organization.[27] A letter sent to the White House by a young student prompted a visit by President Obama.[28]

Conclusion

The first part of this chapter outlined trajectories of the resilience concept in organizational and institutional theory, and thus attempted to shift attention from focusing on only a single point of failure or adverse event, to examining the particular sequence of events and decisions, and, more importantly, potential points of intervention that exist in and for large technical systems and their organizational and institutional environment.

The second part of this chapter outlined a framework for analyzing and managing slow-onset events, from the type of basic human need affected to the type of long-term recovery. The example of the Flint Water Crisis illustrates how this long-term view might be more appropriate for slow-onset events, in particular since conditions similar to those present in Flint, Michigan, can be found all across the U.S.[29] Understanding the complexity and coupling behavior in socio-technical systems, combined with the recognition that, ultimately, all disasters are local, are key to implementing the national policy goal of all-hazards community resilience.

Using the kind of schematic presented here, public managers at the state and local level can track critical developments and their outcomes even without knowing whether they might result in an actual emergency. In addition to assisting in identifying *what* happened (or ought to have happened as a counterfactual), it can also be used to assign *who* made (or ought to have made) the decisions implied in the sequence of events and stages of intervention. A related question of particular importance in public policy is the question of who pays for the implementation of such decisions—the individual household, the municipality, or the utility.

While this type of comprehensive analysis is already part of scenarios or table-top exercises, an increased focus on day-to-day decisions affecting the quality of vital services and infrastructures in a community can only be beneficial for the core mission of both regulators, city managers and emergency responders, which is ensuring health, safety, and security of all citizens.

Notes

1. For a taxonomy and terminology of different types of disasters, see e.g., TF QCDM/WADEM. "Health Disaster Management: Guidelines for Evaluation and Research in the "Utstein Style." *Prehosp Disast Med* 17 (Suppl 3) (2002): 31–55. [Task Force on Quality Control of Disaster Management (TFQCDM); World Association for Disaster and Emergency Medicine (WADEM)].

2. See e.g., Kevin Smith, *Environmental Hazards: Assessing Risk and Reducing Disaster* (London: Routledge, 2009).

3. U.S. Department of Homeland Security. *National Infrastructure Protection Plan (NIPP)* (Washington, D.C.: U.S. Department of Homeland Security, 2013).

4. U.S. Department of Homeland Security. *National Incident Management System (NIMS)* (Washington, D.C.: U.S. Department of Homeland Security, 2008).

5. The National Planning Frameworks are part of the National Preparedness System, with one national framework document for each of the five preparedness mission areas designated to support the goals of the 2011 Presidential Policy Directive/PPD-8: National Preparedness: Prevention, Protection, Mitigation, Response, and Disaster Recovery. See U.S. Federal Emergency Management Agency. "National Planning Frameworks." Accessed April 19, 2016. http://www.fema.gov/national-planning-frameworks.

6. Charles Perrow, *Normal Accidents: Living with High-Risk Technologies*. New York: Basic Books, 1984.

7. "Normal" accident is thus a bit misleading; it does not refer to the frequency of failures and is different from every day or routine accidents like car crashes. It refers to accidents being a normal aspect of a system's particular level of complexity and coupling. In other words: death is a normal part of life, but everyone dies only once.

8. Perrow, 1984, 70. Clearly, this eliminates a large number of causes for system failures, and doesn't even mention intentional sabotage or attacks. He also explicitly excludes so-called "final accidents" that completely destroy a system, for example a dam hit by an earthquake.

9. In what could be called the "glass half full" version of Perrow's "glass half empty" view of system failure, there is a body of work that asserts that certain organizational structures can contribute significantly to the prevention of disasters. Interestingly, these so-called high-reliability organizations (HRO) often coincide with high-risk environments such as nuclear power plants and ships. They are characterized by high levels of technical competence and sustained performance, rewards for error discovery and correction, decentralized authority patterns, structural redundancy, and adequate and reliable funding. For further reading, see e.g., Todd. R. LaPorte, and Chris Thomas. "Regulatory Compliance and the Ethos of Quality Enhancement: Surprises in Nuclear Power Plant Operations." *Journal of Public Administration Research and Theory* 5 (1994): 250-295; Paul Schulman, Emery Roe, Michael van Eeten, and Mark de Bruijne. "High Reliability and the Management of Critical Infrastructures." *Journal of Contingencies and Crisis Management* 12, no. 1 (March 2004): 14–28. doi: 10.1111/j.0966-0879.2004.01201003.x

10. Those planning documents contain a mix of best practices, examples, organizational directives, resources, and management suggestions for coordinating federal, state, and local authorities, and private sector entities to plan, prevent,

response and recover in the case of incidents of national significance (U.S. Department of Homeland Security, 2008; 2010).

11. Louise K. Comfort, "Managing Intergovernmental Responses to Terrorism and Other Extreme Events." *Publius* 32, no. 4 (2002): 29–40.

12. Louise K. Comfort, "Risk and Resilience: Inter-Organizational Learning Following the Northridge Earthquake of 17 January 1994." *Journal of Contingencies and Crisis Management* 2(3) (1994): 157–170.

13. Patricia H. Longstaff, "Security, Resilience, and Communication in Unpredictable Environments Such as Terrorism, Natural Disasters, and Complex Technology." *Center for Information Policy Research.* Cambridge, MA: Harvard University, 2005; Patricia H. Longstaff, Nicholas J. Armstrong, Keli Perrin, Whitney May Parker, and Matthew A. Hidek. "Building Resilient Communities: A Preliminary Framework for Assessment." *Homeland Security Affairs* 6, no. 3 (2010).

14. Longstaff, 2005, 25.

15. Aaron Wildavsky, *Searching for Safety*. New Brunswick, NJ: Transaction Books, 1988.

16. Wildavsky uses the terms danger and damage instead of threat and consequence when analyzing risk. "Anticipation is a mode of control by a central mind; efforts are made to predict and prevent potential dangers before damage is done ... Resilience is the capacity to cope with unanticipated dangers after they have become manifest, learning to bounce back. ... Anticipation seeks to preserve stability: the less fluctuation, the better. Resilience accommodates variability; one may not do so well in good times but learn to persist in the bad."

17. Adapted from: Christoph Hohenemser, Robert W. Kates, and Paul Slovic. "The Nature of Technological Hazard." *Science* 220 (1983): 378–84; and Keith Smith, 2009, 13.

18. U.S. Department of Homeland Security. *Water Sector-Specific* Plan. *An Annex to the National Infrastructure Protection Plan*. Washington, D.C., 2010.

19. Steven M. Rinaldi, James P. Peerenboom, and Terrence K. Kelly. "Identifying, Understanding, and Analyzing Critical Infrastructure Interdependencies." *IEEE Control Systems Magazine* 21, no. 6 (2001): 11–25.

20. Jennifer Dixon, "How Flint's Water Crisis Unfolded." *Detroit Free Press.* Accessed April 26, 2016. http://www.freep.com/pages/interactives/flint-water-crisis-timeline/

21. Ibid.

22. For example, drinking water contaminated with methane was observed in parts of Pennsylvania and Texas, and linked to nearby shale gas extraction (fracking). While this has been indicated in other communities, it turns out that in this case, faulty well integrity, such as poor casing and cementing, was the primary cause. This case also highlights the importance of pursuing alternative explanations or counterfactuals in risk analysis. See Thomas H. Darrah, Avner Vengosh, Robert B. Jackson, Nathaniel R. Warner and Robert J. Poreda. "Noble Gases Identify the Mechanisms of Fugitive Gas Contamination in Drinking-Water Wells Overlying the Marcellus and Barnett Shales." *Proceedings of the National Academy of Sciences.* September 15, 2014. Accessed April 20, 2016. http://www.pnas.org/cgi/doi/10.1073/pnas.1322107111.

23. Alison Young, "Some States, Utilities Balk at Disclosing Locations of Lead Water Pipes." *USA Today*, April 21, 2016. Accessed April 24, 2016. http://www.usatoday.com/story/news/2016/04/21/lead-water-service-line-location-transparency/83201228/.

24. Dixon, 2016.

25. U.S. House Committee on Oversight and Government Reform. *Examining Federal Administration of the Safe Drinking Water Act in Flint, Michigan.* Washington, D.C., 2016. https://oversight.house.gov/hearing/examining-federal-administration-of-the-safe-drinking-water-act-in-flint-michigan/.

26. Since the 2014 switch, lead was not the only contaminant observed; coliform bacteria (e-coli), trihalomethanes (THMs), and possibly legionella bacteria (Legionnaires' disease) were present at different times as well.

27. Associated Press. "Mom in Center of Flint Water Crisis Starts Nonprofit." *Detroit Free Press*, April 26, 2016. http://www.freep.com/story/news/local/michigan/flint-water-crisis/2016/04/26/flint-water-crisis-leeanne-walters-nonprofit/83534206/.

28. Keith Laing, and Chad Livengood. "Child's Letter Stirs Obama's Visit to Flint." *The Detroit News*, April 28, 2016. http://www.detroitnews.com/story/news/michigan/flint-water-crisis/2016/04/27/obama-visit-flint-spotlight-water-crisis/83590046/.

29. By some estimates, one in five census tracts in older urban areas such as New York and Chicago have very high risks of lead exposure, and still one in ten census tracts in younger urban areas such as Los Angeles. The census tracts for these estimates were identified using the U.S. Census Bureau 2010-2014 American Community Survey 5-Year Estimates on poverty and age of housing. See Sarah Frostenson and Sarah Kliff, "The risk of lead poisoning isn't just in Flint. So we mapped the risk in every neighborhood in America." Accessed April 16, 2016. http://www.vox.com/a/lead-exposure-risk-map.

CHAPTER 7

FLINT AND THE INFLUENCE OF INSTITUTIONAL RELATIONSHIPS ON POLICY CHANGE DURING FOCUSING EVENTS

Jennifer F. Sklarew

Introduction

Many analyses have examined how various authorities' actions led to the water crisis in Flint, Michigan. Institutional relationships offer a lens to examine how this puzzling trajectory developed. Shedding light on the potential for meaningful policy and regulatory change, one can look to the changes in relationships, including relationships that stayed "status quo" between the federal, state, and local governments and local residents after the crisis. Analysis of government documents related to the events that unfolded in Flint reveal that relationships between the U.S. Environmental Protection Agency (EPA). state regulators at the Michigan Department of Environmental Quality (MDEQ) and officials in the Governor's office and the Michigan Department of Health and Human Services (DHHS), local officials in the Flint City Council, Flint Public Works and Genesee County, and Flint residents played influential roles in the creation and handling of the crisis. Understanding how the crisis has affected these institutional relationships illuminates the challenges facing the policy and regulatory transformation needed to avert future crises.

The Role of Institutions in Public Policy Frameworks

New institutionalism and policy process frameworks both highlight the importance of institutions in catalyzing or thwarting policy change after crises. New institutionalists such as Paul Pierson, Peter Hall, Kathleen Thelen, and James Mahoney view institutions as dynamic and evolving through a process of creation and change. This is influenced by generations of actors' interactions.[1] Policy process theorists like John Kingdon and Thomas Birkland highlight the role of institutions in driving critical junctures that can emerge from focusing events.[2]

The concept of focusing events initiated by Kingdon, and elaborated upon by Birkland and others, involves focusing events that occur during brief time periods. These events provide a catalyst and opportunity for change. Kingdon depicts focusing events—such as crises or disasters —as mechanisms that push problems to the forefront. Thus opening "policy windows" to create a critical juncture that can lead to policy change. Followers of Kingdon and Pierson differ on the time frame and precipitating factors behind these critical junctures. Kingdon and other policy process scholars note specific points in time when external shocks become critical junctures that punctuate a stable system. Institutionalists frame critical junctures as phases that can range from days to a decade, rather than one-time occurrences pinpointed on a calendar. These phases can include a focusing event, however still driven by institutions and the shifts in them over time. This leads to gradual change in established paths.[3]

The Flint Water Crisis seems to embody the focusing event described by Kingdon and other policy process theorists, accompanied by the institutional changes depicted by historical institutionalists. Joining these new institutionalist and policy process frameworks thus offers a helpful perspective on the ways in which institutional relationships contributed to creation of a focusing event in Flint. Combining these two frameworks also enables analysis of how these relationships and changes in them have influenced the crisis' potential of becoming a critical juncture that elicits long-term policy change.

Birkland and some other scholars of the policy process suggest that focusing events alone may not engender policy action, and action from within the policy community must support the effect of such events in order to make them focal.[4] Birkland highlights the degree of organization and polarization within the policy community as factors affecting the impact of focusing events on policy change. These features identified by Birkland contribute to a broader concept of power balance—or clout—and cooperation/conflict across groups in the policy community.

Documents from the various government agencies, the Flint Water Advisory Task Force, and the media reveal that several key relationships contributed to the Flint Water Crisis. These same relationships will shape *if and how* long-term policy change emerges. These relationships include: those between federal and state regulators; federal and state regulators and the Flint residents; and the local government's relationships with the state government, the water utility agency, and the Flint residents. Analyzing the levels of cooperation and trust in these relationships and the relative clout across these groups as the crisis unfolded helps to explain the actions that created the focusing event. Shifts in this trust, cooperation, and clout across these groups also affect the potential for policy and regulatory change emerging from the crisis.

The Role of Relationships in the Flint Crisis

I. Local and State Government

Cooperation and trust are necessary for the smooth functioning of governmental agencies and development and implementation of effective policies and regulations. However, the Flint Water Crisis reflects the ways in which superficial cooperation and trust can hinder recognition of a public health and safety concern that transcends expectations. Ambiguous authority can compound this effect, as demonstrated by the influence of Flint's local and state officials' perceptions of responsibility during the crisis. This ineffective cooperation, distrust, and confusion over clout can hinder the potential for effective state and federal policy transformation to prevent future crises.

Decline in Superficial Cooperation and Trust. As Flint shifted its water supply to the Flint River, superficial cooperation and trust characterized the relationship between local and state governments. This surface cooperation and trust focused on compliance with existing regulations and policies, rather than the shared goal of public safety and health protection. An MDEQ document from November 2015 reflects this relationship: "The DEQ had no reason to question the validity of the City's reports until the DEQ heard City employees revealing to the media that the City did not know for certain if its compliance monitoring was collected from homes with lead service lines."[5] Assumptions of compliance with existing regulations discouraged recognition of potential safety and health threats. These assumptions also created an environment that limited enforcement and verification of such compliance. December 23, 2015 responses from the State Office of the Auditor General reflect this problem: "DEQ did not verify that only tier 1 sample sites were selected. DEQ relies on the Flint [Water Treatment Plant's] certification of sample sites and does not perform any independent verification of those certifications."[6]

Local officials in Flint similarly trusted Michigan's state regulators and officials, despite rising conflict. In a February 2016 media interview, former Mayor Dayne Walling said of the state-appointed emergency manager, "Even though we disagreed on many things ... I fundamentally trusted that it would be done right. That was a mistake."[7] Former Flint emergency manager Darnell Earley, appointed by the state, asserts that he relied on state and federal experts to provide accurate technical information on lead leaching into the water supply, but he received no such information for months after the switch to the Flint River.[8] The Flint Water Advisory Task Force's final report notes that "Flint Public Works acted on inaccurate and improper guidance from MDEQ."[9] The report also criticizes MDEQ's poor enforcement of regulatory requirements city officials should have followed.

As the crisis progressed, superficial cooperation and trust turned to conflict. Throughout 2015, Genesee County Environmental Health Supervisor Jim Henry argued with MDEQ and MDHHS officials over the Flint River water's role in the Legionnaire's outbreak. E-mail exchanges reflect this disagreement and state officials' refusal to investigate Henry's suspicions of a linkage. Henry contacted federal agencies and was later chastised by state officials for bypassing them and ignoring protocol.[10] In March 2016, Mayor Karen Weaver filed notice of the city's right to sue the state for the crisis, indicating continuation of conflict between local and state governments. Ambiguous delineation of authority contributed to this decline in cooperation and trust.

Confusion over Clout. The relative clout of state and local governments remained unclear throughout the crisis, contributing to it and thwarting rapid resolution. Several conflicting indicators reflect this ambiguous authority. The Flint Water Advisory Task Force's final report, released in March 2016, cites the state's appointment of Flint's emergency manager as one of the first contributors to the crisis:

> The Flint Water Crisis occurred when state-appointed emergency managers replaced local representative decision-making in Flint, removing the checks and balances and public accountability that come with public decision-making. Emergency managers made key decisions that contributed to the crisis, from the use of the Flint River to delays in reconnecting to the DWSD once water quality problems were encountered.[11]

Next, the state treasurer, Andy Dillon, approved the emergency manager's decision to switch the city's water supply to the Flint River. Former

Flint water treatment plant supervisor Mike Glasgow cites instructions from MDEQ engineer Mike Prysby as the reason corrosion controls were not implemented at the plant prior to the switch. Prysby apparently told Glasgow that a year of water testing was required prior to implementation of corrosion controls. Glasgow did not agree, but he did not object.[12]

In contrast, state officials and regulators cited the city as responsible for the crisis. Under the 1976 Michigan Safe Drinking Water Act (PA 399), the City of Flint is responsible for treating drinking water, as well as testing it for specified contaminants and reporting the results to the MDEQ to verify that the samples meet federal and state standards.[13] MDEQ officials have posited that they based their actions on assumptions that city authorities were conducting sampling complaint with regulations. In a September 2015 e-mail, the Governor's Chief of Staff, Dennis Muchmore, told Governor Snyder that the "DEQ and DCH feel that some in Flint are taking the very sensitive issue of children's exposure to lead and trying to turn it into a political football claiming the departments are underestimating the impacts on the populations and particularly trying to shift responsibility to the state." He continues on, "I can't figure out why the state is responsible except that Dillon did make the ultimate decision so we're not able to avoid the subject. The real responsibility rests with the county, city and Karegnondi Water Authority (KWA), but since the issue here is the health of citizens and their children we're taking a proactive approach putting MDHHS out there as an educator."[14] In another e-mail to the Governor the next day, Muchmore expresses a similar view, along with frustration over divergent perceptions of responsibility for and management of the crisis: "Of course, some of the Flint people respond by looking for someone to blame instead of working to reduce anxiety. We can't tolerate increased lead levels in any event, but it's really the city's water system that needs to deal with it. We're throwing as much assistance as possible at the lead problem as regardless of what the levels, explanations or proposed solutions, the residents and particularly the poor need help to deal with it."[15] December 2015 responses from Michigan's Office of the Auditor General corroborate this view of city leadership, noting that since MDEQ does not oversee the Flint water treatment plant, the state regulator has no accountability measures to ensure correct sampling protocols and "relies on Flint's certification of sample sites."[16]

In a December 7, 2015 letter to the Governor, the Flint Water Advisory Task Force highlights the need for better coordination of responsibilities across all levels of government: "One primary concern we have at this point is that the current efforts appear to be taking place in the absence of a larger project coordination framework that measures results and clearly delineates responsibilities for continuing actions to protect public health." The Task Force also recommended that the state government lead this coordination, stating in the letter, "We believe the state is best positioned to facilitate this larger framework."[17] In a December 29, 2015 letter and in its final report, the Task Force ultimately assigned responsibility for the crisis to state regulators. The letter states that "[a]lthough many individuals and entities at state and local levels contributed to creating and prolonging the problem, MDEQ is the government agency that has responsibility to ensure safe drinking water in Michigan. It failed in that responsibility and must be held accountable for that failure."[18] This criticism reveals a need for broader policy change to clarify responsibility for water safety and health oversight and action.

The state government's relationship with the local government reflects superficial and waning cooperation and trust as the Flint Water Crisis unfolded. This problematic relationship, coupled with confusion over clout, contributed to creation and protraction of the crisis. It also complicates transformation of the crisis into a critical juncture that can lead to meaningful policy change beyond replacement of specific individuals.

II. State Government and Federal Government

The state regulator's relationship with the federal government parallels the relationship with the local government. Once again, superficial cooperation and trust, combined with perceptions of overlapping jurisdiction, contributed to and slowed resolution of the Flint Water Crisis.

Decline in Surface Cooperation and Trust in Compliance. Government documents and comments from EPA officials reflect a state-federal regulator relationship characterized by a lack of true cooperation, coupled with declining trust. The EPA trusted that the MDEQ was interpreting regulations in ways intended to protect citizens, while the MDEQ focused on compliance with these regulations. As an example, while asserting compliance in a February 27, 2015 e-mail to EPA officials, MDEQ's Stephen Busch stated that "the City of Flint ... has an optimized corrosion control program and conducts quarterly water quality parameter monitoring at 25 sites and has not had any unusual results."[19] The EPA assumed that the program included corrosion controls, while subsequent MDEQ documents assert that officials were referring to water testing to determine the need for controls. A November 3, 2015 EPA memo acknowledges the ambiguity of the federal guideline and provides clarification; however, later the clarification is criticized by the Flint Water Advisory Task Force as unnecessary. These exchanges reflect an effort to continue surface cooperation focused on compliance, rather than safety and health.[20]

Other actions by the state regulators also embodied surface cooperation with federal regulators. These actions included MDEQ guidance to Flint citizens that included flushing of taps prior to sampling, as well as MDEQ's discarding of two high-lead water samples based on an interpretation of federal guidelines that prioritized compliance over safety and health. EPA officials conflicted with MDEQ officials over both of these actions, prompting compliance-based justifications from state officials, as well as state requests for federal clarifications of the guidelines. E-mail messages from EPA Region 5 Regulations Manager Miguel Del Toral as early as February 2015 question these actions, reflecting conflict between federal and state agencies.[21] Del Toral's later correspondences highlight the superficial cooperation between the EPA and the MDEQ, noting coordination across local, state, and federal agencies to publicly minimize the perceptions of a lead threat in Flint.[22]

The MDEQ's focus on compliance with federal regulations, rather than the promotion of safety, weakened the EPA's trust and reflected superficial cooperation. The Flint Water Advisory Task Force's final report accuses the MDEQ of waiting "months before accepting [the] EPA's offer to engage its lead (Pb) experts to help address the Flint water situation," adding that "at times, MDEQ staff were dismissive and unresponsive."[23] Although the federal agency did not take formal action challenging the state's handling of the crisis until November 2015, when the EPA announced an audit of Michigan's drinking water program; the EPA's correspondences with MDEQ in 2015 reflect increasing conflict behind the scenes. Numerous documented e-mails and phone calls between EPA Region 5 officials and MDEQ officials include disagreements over sampling techniques, optimized corrosion controls, and whether the situation required government action.

The conflict between federal and state regulators ultimately culminated in the EPA's emergency order issued in January 2016, in which the EPA states that "[t]he City, MDEQ, and the State have failed to take adequate measures to protect public health ... there continue to be delays in responding to critical EPA recommendations and in implementing the actions necessary to reduce and minimize the presence of lead and other contaminants in the water supply both now and in the future."[24] Even the EPA's order and MDEQ's change in leadership did not return the federal-state relationship to cooperation. The conflict has continued, including arguments over compliance. In a January 22 letter responding to the EPA's emergency order, new MDEQ Director Keith Creagh asserts that "although the Order states that the State has failed to take adequate measures to comply with the USEPA's demands, to our knowledge, the State has complied with every recent demand or request made by the USEPA."[25] This continued conflict over compliance at the expense of safety cooperation hinders creation of a critical juncture that advances resolution and triggers policy change to prevent future crises. As the crisis has continued, conflict between federal and state regulators has expanded to include a battle over clout.

Strategic Ceding of Clout. Paralleling the state-local government relationship, state and federal regulators have engaged in a battle over responsibility for and authority to resolve Flint's water crisis. Just as they cited local responsibility for the water crisis, Michigan's state officials also have noted federal responsibility for state oversight. However, Michigan's state government officially maintains responsibility for safe drinking water across the state. Under the cooperative federalism framework of the federal Safe Drinking Water Act, states can apply for primacy, or authority to implement the Act, and the Michigan state government has maintained primacy since 1976. Primacy requires that the state adopt and enforce standards at least as stringent as the federal Act.

As the federal regulator, the EPA is responsible for annually evaluating Michigan's program to ensure compliance with federal standards. The EPA also has the authority to supersede a state's primacy by invoking Section 1431 of the Act based on information that a contaminant is threatening the state's drinking water supply. Instead of assuming control of Flint's water supply safety, the EPA continued to urge state regulators to take action. In Congressional testimony, the EPA's former Region 5 Administrator, Susan Hedman, cites constraints on the EPA's clout as the reason for deferring to the state: "And, while I used the threat of enforcement action to motivate the state and city to move forward, we found that the enforcement options available to us were of limited utility last fall, due to the unique circumstances of this case."[26] The EPA ordered an audit of the MDEQ's program in November 2015 to determine compliance with the Safe Drinking Water Act. The Flint Water Advisory Task Force's final report acknowledges the state's primacy and responsibility, but it also criticizes the EPA's delayed enforcement of the Safe Drinking Water Act and Lead and Copper Rule as "prolonging the calamity."[27] The Task Force condemns this failure to exert clout, even criticizing the EPA's November 3 memo as reflective of EPA's deference to state regulators.[28]

The federal agency's January 2016 emergency order assuming responsibility for water testing in Flint came after many months of documented discussions among EPA officials about the lead concern and doubts over the state's effective handling of it.[29] Despite the emergency order, conflict over federal vs. state clout continues. MDEQ's response to the order challenges the EPA's legal authority to mandate state actions: "From a legal perspective, we also question whether the USEPA has the legal authority to order a State and its agencies to take the actions outlined in the Order."[30] In its January 24, 2016 response, the EPA states, "We do not agree with the issues you raise about the Agency's legal authority."[31] The Flint Water Advisory Task Force's criticism of both state and federal regulators highlights the problems created by poor coordination and unclear leadership roles. In conjunction with conflict and distrust, these problems have thwarted resolution of the crisis and challenged creation of a critical juncture that elicits policy and regulatory change. Even if policy change were to occur, perpetuation of conflict and unclear authority to implement policies and regulations would weaken their effectiveness.

Local Government and Public

Public conflict with and distrust in the government can catalyze transformation of crises into critical junctures. While citizens have relatively less clout than government officials in the policymaking process, distrust and conflict can galvanize public pressure for policy change. This scenario has emerged in Flint, but the other relationships described here also determine whether true policy change will materialize.

Shattering of Cooperation and Trust. When the local government announced the switch to the Flint River, Flint citizens cooperated with and trusted in the government to protect public health and safety. Government communication on the background for the switch and assurances of minimal risk garnered this public support. An April 25, 2014 press release from the City of Flint heralds the switch and explains that "[e]ach temporary stint on local water proved three things to city employees and residents alike: That a transition to local river water could be done seamlessly, and that it was both sensible and safe for us to use our own water as a primary water source in Flint."[32] The press release acknowledges public concern over water quality and reassures residents that testing has proven the potability of Flint River water:

> Even with a proven track record of providing perfectly good water for Flint, there still remains lingering uncertainty about the quality of the water. In an effort to dispel myths and promote the truth about the Flint River and its viability as a residential water resource, there have been numerous studies and tests conducted on its water by several different independent organizations. In addition to what has been found in independent studies, it is also the responsibility of the City of Flint Water Service Center to continually test the water provided to city residents.[33]

State government officials also promoted public trust and cooperation. The same press release quotes MDEQ's Michael Prysby as verifying that "the quality of the water being put out meets all of our drinking water standards and Flint water is safe to drink."[34] These government assertions assuaged public concern over the safety of water from the Flint River. The Flint River Watershed Coalition also invited city residents to participate in monitoring exercises in spring 2014 "to gain firsthand knowledge in the health and vitality of our Flint River."[35] This inclusion of citizens in the sampling process deepened trust in the government and promoted cooperation.

However, as citizens began to notice health problems and physical differences in their water, their trust in local and state governments declined. When affected residents like Lee-Anne Walters raised questions, they received assurances from MDEQ that testing did not reveal lead problems in the water. In a February 2016 Congressional hearing, Walters testified, "We fought with the city and the state that something was wrong and we were dismissed."[36] EPA's Del Toral's interim report, which ascribed Flint's high lead levels to the city's water pipes, became public in July 2015, furthering distrust in city and state officials' communications to Flint residents. The EPA's subsequent apology to city officials for releasing the report before it was "revised and fully vetted by EPA management" widened public distrust in the government to include EPA.[37] And yet, Flint residents continued to cooperate with government instructions for water testing, including the pre-flushing of taps later determined to have artificially lowered lead readings.

By fall 2015, Flint residents' trust in the government's ability to promote public safety and health had eroded completely. Media coverage of the crisis widened this effect, as accounts of government misinformation reached citizens across the nation. The city government's simultaneous efforts to release information and placate the public deepened distrust. A September 25, 2015 lead advisory press release offers an example, as it asserts full compliance with the Safe Drinking Water Act while contradicting previously released information by acknowledging the presence of lead in Flint's drinking water. The press release frames the advisory as an educational tool and implicitly suggests that Flint's lead levels may not be high.[38] In a September 26, 2015 e-mail to the Governor, Muchmore summarized, "The residents are caught in a swirl of misinformation and long-term distrust of local government unlikely to be resolved."[39]

Public perceptions of uncooperative government responses contributed to the decline in public trust and escalation of conflict between Flint citizens and the government. As the crisis unfolded, MDEQ and MDHHS conflicted with local organizations over validity of sampling for lead in water and blood. A September 2015 e-mail to MDEQ and Governor's office staff from Geraldine Lasher, MDHHS Deputy Director of External Relations and Communications, demonstrates state agencies' challenging of local independent investigations: "MDHHS epidemiologists continue to review the 'data' provided by a Hurley hospital physician that showed an increase in lead activity following the change in water supply. While we continue to review this data, we have stated publicly that Hurley conducted their analysis in a much different way than we do at the department."[40]

This disagreement over methods delayed policy action to remedy the problems with Flint's water. The Flint Water Advisory Task Force's December 29 letter to Governor Snyder recognizes that state agencies "might disagree with the opinions of others on a variety of issues, including testing protocol, interpretation of testing results, the requirements of federal law and rules, and other matters."[41] The Task Force criticizes both MDEQ and MDHHS for their approach to this conflict, asserting that "[i]n fact, the MDEQ seems to have been more determined to discredit the work of others, who ultimately proved to be right, than to pursue its own oversight responsibility."[42] The letter highlights the "failure in tone and substance of MDEQ response to the public," asserting that "[t]hroughout 2015, as the public raised concerns and as independent studies and testing were conducted and brought to the attention of MDEQ, the agency's response was often one of aggressive dismissal, belittlement, and attempts to discredit these efforts and the individuals involved."[43] In its final report, the Task Force again criticizes state regulators for prolonging the crisis by promoting conflict through attempts to discredit others' data that reflected water problems, as well through reluctance to share their own data on lead levels in blood and water.[44]

Public distrust of and conflict with government officials has hindered resolution of the crisis. As the Task Forces notes in their December 29 letter, "The current level of distrust ... serves to compromise the effective delivery of protected services designed to address ongoing public health issues."[45] The letter also highlights the problematic role of ambiguous clout across government agencies in contributing to this distrust and conflict, stressing that "[e]stablishing responsibility and accountability is the first step in re-establishing the trust between the citizens of Flint and their government and the agencies whose responsibility it is to protect their health."[46] Even attempts to demonstrate government cooperation have failed to restore public trust in the government's ability to promote water safety and health. Flint residents responded skeptically to February 2016 water testing by teams from federal, state, and local agencies, indicating that they would not trust any data produced by the government, nor do they trust that existing regulations will protect them.[47] While the testing shows a decline in residential water lead levels, more than 600 homes' test results still reveal lead levels above the EPA's action level. One such resident, Fortina Harris, declared to CNN in March, "You can't trust the government. Their trust gone down the Flint River."[48] A class action lawsuit filed in February 2016 against state and local officials reflects ongoing conflict.

This loss of trust spurred Flint citizens and others to take matters into their own hands, shifting clout from the government to the public in the context of data collection and analysis.

Shift Toward Public Demand for Clout. The Flint crisis initially featured government clout over the public. The government controlled the information citizens received, and the public had little influence on regulations and policies governing water safety and the switch to Flint River water. The Flint Water Advisory Task Force found that "[t]he emergency manager structure made it extremely difficult for Flint citizens to alter or check decision-making on preparations for use of Flint River water, or to receive responses to concerns about subsequent water quality issues."[49] Even after problems emerged; government agencies conducted the sampling, analyzed the results, interpreted the regulations, and determined the course and pace of action, all without public input.

However, Flint residents' increasing conflict with and distrust of the government led to public demand for clout. A grassroots movement to gain control of water sampling and analysis emerged. Residents shared these findings with other residents, as well as government officials, and then ultimately, the media. The Task Force highlighted this shift toward public control as one of the key factors catalyzing resolution of the water crisis:

> The Flint Water Crisis is also a story, however, of something that did work: the critical role played by engaged Flint citizens, by individuals both inside and outside of government who had the expertise and willingness to question and challenge government leadership, and by members of a free press who used the tools that enable investigative journalism. Without their courage and persistence, this crisis likely never would have been brought to light and mitigation efforts never begun.[50]

As Flint residents found that their data confirmed a problem denied by government officials, their distrust in existing infrastructure and regulations grew. Lee-Anne Walters' testimony reflects this distrust, coupled with continued city and state government efforts to control public knowledge of and influence on water safety regulations. The testimony describes meetings with city and state officials, in which Walters was told that the interim report by EPA's Del Toral "was flawed, and there would be no final report."[51] Walters shifted public clout by releasing the interim report to the media.

This shift toward public control over knowledge of water safety led Flint residents to demand that the government replace lead service lines. The city government's resulting request for state funds to implement the line replacement reflects increased public clout at the local level. Flint Mayor Karen Weaver told the media that "... in order for us to build trust back in the government, and trust back in the water, we've got to have new pipes."[52] And yet, the state government's $58 million pledge to Flint does not include funds allocated for line replacement, reflecting continuation of state officials' clout over local government and the public regarding infrastructure changes.

Distrust in all levels of government and the existing regulatory system spurred Flint citizens to press for more clout in decision-making on water infrastructure, as well as water safety regulations and policies, moving the Flint crisis toward a critical juncture.

Influence on Policy Changes to Prevent Future Crises

The focusing event in Flint is forming a critical juncture, but will it result in infrastructure change, regulatory and policy change, both, or neither? The unfolding of the crisis revealed the influence of relationships between the local, state, and federal government and the public. Changes in relationships, including relationships that continue with the status quo, can influence the policy outcomes emerging from facilitated focusing events.

Throughout the crisis, the state government wielded clout over the local and federal government, but deferred action on the Flint Water Crisis as a local problem. While superficial cooperation and trust initially characterized intragovernmental relationships, true cooperation and coordination did not occur. This lack of cooperation between federal, state, and local government agencies contributed to the crisis and was exacerbated by it. Such ineffective cooperation can hinder policy change to resolve it and prevent future crises. In addition, state clout has continued to thwart changes to infrastructure, regulation and policy. The Michigan state government has rejected the local government's calls for state funding to replace lead service lines, as well as proposed federal regulatory and policy changes. These changes would modify the policy empowering state officials to appoint local emergency managers and revise the EPA's authority to enforce the Lead and Copper Rule and Safe Drinking Water Act.

Local and state government clout over the public also contributed to the crisis, despite growing conflict. Disintegration of public trust in local and state officials led to an increase in public clout over information gathering and release, but not changes in infrastructure, policy or regulation. To date, local and state government officials appear to remain focused on rebuilding trust through the quickest, least costly solutions. These measures have not yet improved public trust or reduced conflict. If implemented, replacement of lead service lines could rebuild public trust in the safety of Flint's water. However, this infrastructure change won't likely rebuild trust in the government's ability to oversee public safety and health.

At the federal level, Congressional hearings have elevated the clout of Flint citizens and the researchers assisting them, offering an opportunity to share their data and analyses, as well as their views on changes needed to prevent similar crises in the future. Whether this increase in public clout results in broader lasting change remains to be seen.

Lessons for the Future: Fixing Water and Governance Systems

Calls to address the crisis in Flint have moved beyond local fixes. They also transcend the water system to address the governance system. The Flint Water Advisory Task Force and those who have testified before Congress have offered recommendations for policy changes to improve the effectiveness of the Lead and Copper Rule and the Safe Drinking Water Act. Several pieces of federal legislation introduced in 2016 would impose regulatory changes to empower the EPA and the public. The proposed measures include requiring the EPA to notify residents and health departments when a state fails to notify them of lead levels in water requiring action. The bills also shift clout from local and state governments to the federal government by imbuing the EPA with responsibility for releasing results from lead monitoring.[53] Many of these changes suggest that protecting public safety and health requires institutional shifts that promote true cooperation, trust and a balance of clout across levels of government and the public.

Promoting True Cooperation. Rather than promoting regulatory compliance as a goal, policies and regulations should emphasize cooperation to promote safety and health. Compliance should be one means of achieving this goal. Such a shift would foster true cooperation aimed at promoting safety, while minimizing conflict over technicalities.

Fostering Trust through Transparency. Building trust requires transparency of the regulatory and policy process, not just transparency of the results of the process. Coupled with cooperation on safety and health goals that transcend compliance, this transparency can empower all actors to participate in achieving these goals.

Achieving Clout Balance and Clarity. Effective protection of safety and health requires clear delineation of responsibilities and clout across levels of government, as well as empowerment of the public in the policymaking and implementation process. Such clout balance and clarity would reduce conflict over authority and responsibility, avoiding some crises and catalyzing critical junctures to empower timely resolution of others.

Not Just Water under the Bridge

The Flint Water Crisis is creating a critical juncture for policies and regulations that protect public water safety and health. Policy and regulatory changes to prevent future crises must address more than water infrastructure. They also must extend beyond minor regulatory tweaks, striving to shape the institutional relationships that influence their effectiveness. Lasting, meaningful change that protects public safety and health will promote cooperation, trust and balance in these relationships.

Notes

1. Paul Pierson, *Politics in Time: History, Institutions, and Social Analysis.* First Edition (Princeton, NJ: Princeton University Press, 2004); James Mahoney and Kathleen Thelen, *Explaining Institutional Change: Ambiguity, Agency, and Power,* 1st ed. (New York: Cambridge University Press, 2009).

2. John Kingdon, *Agendas, Alternatives, and Public Policies.* 2nd ed. (New York: Addison-Wesley Educational Publishers, Inc., 1997); Thomas Birkland, *After Disaster: Agenda Setting, Public Policy, and Focusing Events* (Washington, D.C.: Georgetown University Press, 1997).

3. Peter Hall and Kathleen Thelen, "Institutional Change in Varieties of Capitalism." *Socio-Economic Review* 7 (1): 7–34, 2009; James Mahoney and Kathleen Thelen, *Explaining Institutional Change: Ambiguity, Agency, and Power,* 1st ed. (New York: Cambridge University Press, 2009).

4. E.g., Baumgartner, Frank R., and Bryan D. Jones, *Agendas and Instability in American Politics.* First edition (University of Chicago Press, 1993); John Kingdon,

Agendas, Alternatives, and Public Policies. 2nd ed. (New York: Addison-Wesley Educational Publishers, Inc., 1997); Thomas Birkland, *After Disaster: Agenda Setting, Public Policy, and Focusing Events* (Washington, D.C.: Georgetown University Press, 1997); Christoph Stefes and Frank N. Laird, "Creating Path Dependency: The Divergence of German and US Renewable Energy Policy," *SSRN eLibrary*, 2010.

5. Michigan Department of Environmental Quality, City of Flint Drinking Water Outline Prepared by the Michigan Department of Environmental Quality for the Flint Water Task Force, November 16, 2015, 16.

6. Office of the Auditor General, *Additional Questions answered by the OAG*, December 23, 2015.

7. Anna Maria Barry-Jester, "What Went Wrong In Flint," *FiveThirty-Eight.com*, January 26, 2016, accessed on February 12, 2016, http://fivethirtyeight.com/features/what-went-wrong-in-flint-water-crisis-michigan/

8. Earley's predecessor, Ed Kurtz, authorized the switch. Associated Press, "Former EPA Official Defends Actions on Flint Water Crisis," *Associated Press*, March 15, 2016, http://www.nbcnews.com/storyline/flint-water-crisis/former-epa-official-defends-actions-flint-water-crisis-n538946

9. Flint Water Advisory Task Force, *Flint Water Advisory Task Force Final Report*, March 2016, 8.

10. For example, see James Henry, "Email to Jim Collins, Michigan Public Health," June 5, 2015, and Chad Livengood and Karen Bouffard, "Emails: State Mum on Flint Legionnaire's Warning," *The Detroit News*, February 12, 2016.

11. Flint Water Advisory Task Force. *Flint Water Advisory Task Force Final Report.* March 2016, 1.

12. Associated Press. "Flint Official: State Overruled Water Treatment Plan," *NBCNews.com*, March 29, 2016, http://www.nbcnews.com/storyline/flint-water-crisis/flint-official-state-overruled-water-treatment-plan-n547621

13. Michigan Department of Environmental Quality, *City of Flint Drinking Water Outline prepared by the Michigan Department of Environmental Quality for the Flint Water Task Force*, November 16, 2015.

14. Dennis Muchmore, "E-mail to Rick Snyder: Flint water," September 25, 2015.

15. Dennis Muchmore, "E-mail to Rick Snyder: Flint updates," September 26, 2015.

16. Meegan Holland, "E-mail on Office of Auditor General's responses," December 24, 2015.

17. Flint Water Advisory Task Force, *Letter to Governor Snyder*, December 7, 2015.

18. Flint Water Advisory Task Force, *Letter to Governor Snyder*, December 29, 2015.

19. Stephen Busch, Jackson and Lansing District Supervisor, Office of Drinking Water and Municipal Assistance, Department of Environmental Quality, "Email to Miguel Del Toral," February 27, 2015.

20. Peter Grevatt, Director, Office of Ground Water and Drinking Water, Environmental Protection Agency, *Memorandum on Lead and Copper Rule Requirements for Optimal Corrosion Control Treatment for Large Drinking Water Systems*, November 3, 2015.

21. Miguel Del Toral, Environmental Protection Agency, "E-mail to Jennifer Crooks and Mike Prysby, Re: HIGH LEAD: Flint Water testing results," February 27, 2015.

22. Miguel Del Toral, Environmental Protection Agency, "E-mail to Rita Bair, Re: Interim Report on High Lead Levels in Flint," June 25, 2015.

23. Flint Water Advisory Task Force, *Flint Water Advisory Task Force Final Report*, March 2016, 6.

24. Office of Enforcement and Compliance Assurance, Environmental Protection Agency, *Emergency Administrative Order*, January 21, 2016, 8.

25. Keith Creagh, Director, Michigan Department of Environmental Quality, *Letter to Gina McCarthy, Administrator, Environmental Protection Agency*, January 22, 2016.

26. Susan Hedman, "Testimony before House Committee on Oversight and Government Reform" (Washington, DC, March 15, 2016).

27. Flint Water Advisory Task Force, *Flint Water Advisory Task Force Final Report*, March 2016, 1.

28. Flint Water Advisory Task Force, *Flint Water Advisory Task Force Final Report*, March 2016, 9.

29. E.g., Jennifer Crooks, Michigan Program Manager, Drinking Water State Revolving Fund, Environmental Protection Agency, "E-mail to Stephen Busch, HIGH LEAD: FLINT Water testing results," February 26, 2015.

30. Keith Creagh, Director, Michigan Department of Environmental Quality, *Letter to Gina McCarthy, Administrator, Environmental Protection Agency*, January 22, 2016.

31. Mark Pollins, Director of Water Enforcement Division, Environmental Protec-

tion Agency, *Letter to Keith Creagh, Director, Michigan Department of Environmental Quality*, January 24, 2016.

32. Jason Lorenz, *Press Release: City of Flint Officially Begins Using Flint River as Temporary Primary Water Source*, April 25, 2014.

33. Jason Lorenz. *Press Release: City of Flint Officially Begins Using Flint River as Temporary Primary Water Source*, April 25, 2014.

34. Jason Lorenz, *Press Release: City of Flint Officially Begins Using Flint River as Temporary Primary Water Source*, April 25, 2014.

35. Jason Lorenz, *Press Release: City of Flint Officially Begins Using Flint River as Temporary Primary Water Source*, April 25, 2014.

36. Lee-Anne Walters, "Examining Federal Administration of the Safe Drinking Water Act in Flint, Michigan," Testimony before the U.S. House of Representatives Committee on Oversight and Government Reform (Washington, DC, February 3, 2016).

37. Susan Hedman, EPA Region 5 Administrator, "E-mail to Dayne Walling, Re: Comments on Flint Water," July 1, 2015.

38. City of Flint, *Press Release: City of Flint Issues Lead Advisory*, September 25, 2015.

39. Dennis Muchmore, "E-mail to Rick Snyder, Flint updates," September 26, 2015.

40. Geralyn Lasher, "E-mail to Dennis Muchmore, Elizabeth Clement, Nick Lyon, and Dan Wyant, Update," September 25, 2015.

41. Flint Water Advisory Task Force, "Letter to Governor Snyder," December 29, 2015.

42. Flint Water Advisory Task Force, "Letter to Governor Snyder," December 29, 2015.

43. Flint Water Advisory Task Force, "Letter to Governor Snyder," December 29, 2015.

44. Flint Water Advisory Task Force, *Flint Water Advisory Task Force Final Report*, March 2016, 1.

45. Flint Water Advisory Task Force, "Letter to Governor Snyder," December 29, 2015.

46. Flint Water Advisory Task Force, "Letter to Governor Snyder," December 29, 2015.

47. Anna Maria Barry-Jester, "What Went Wrong In Flint," *FiveThirty-Eight.com*, January 26, 2016, http://fivethirtyeight.com/features/what-went-wrong-in-flint-water-crisis-michigan/.

48. Sara Ganim, "Five Months Later in Flint, High Lead Levels Remain," *CNN*, March 5, 2016, http://www.cnn.com/2016/03/04/us/flint-update-five-months-later/

49. Flint Water Advisory Task Force, *Flint Water Advisory Task Force Final Report*, March 2016, 8.

50. Flint Water Advisory Task Force, *Flint Water Advisory Task Force Final Report*, March 2016, 1.

51. Lee-Anne Walters, "Examining Federal Administration of the Safe Drinking Water Act in Flint, Michigan," Testimony before the U.S. House of Representatives Committee on Oversight and Government Reform (Washington, DC, February 3, 2016).

52. Sara Ganim, "Five Months Later in Flint, High Lead Levels Remain," *CNN*, March 5, 2016. http://www.cnn.com/2016/03/04/us/flint-update-five-months-later/

53. Office of Gary Peters, *Press Release: Peters, Stabenow and Kildee to Introduce Public Notification Bill to Prevent Another Flint Water Crisis*, January 27, 2016. In April 2016, Senate Democrats proposed a bill for nationwide line replacement, new requirements for reporting on blood-lead levels and revision of the Lead and Copper Rule that compels the EPA to require lead testing of pipes, establishes household action levels for lead and copper, and improves notification of excessive lead levels. Republican opposition has stalled the bill. Senate Democrats previously proposed a $100 million funding package for Flint in the Water Resources Development Act, also stalled by Republicans in the Senate Environment and Public Works Committee. Before that, funding was included in the Senate energy bill, then removed.

ABOUT THE EDITORS

Tonya E. Thornton (formerly Neaves), Ph.D., is an Assistant Professor and Director of Grants at George Mason University's Schar School of Policy and Government. Tonya's research interests primarily focus on emergency management and community resiliency. Her research has appeared in the *Journal of Emergency Management, Review of Policy Research,* and the *American Journal of Public Health.* She is also an active member of the American Society for Public Administration and is the Treasurer for the Section on Emergency and Crisis Management. Her pragmatic approach is premised on the integration of scholarship with the communities of practice. To date, her research funding approximates $6 million, with expertise in public safety, critical infrastructure, and emergency management.

Andrew D. Williams, AICP, is the co-founder and chief executive officer for The Berkley Group. Previously, he spent over a decade in the public sector in Virginia localities focusing on planning and public works and was responsible for overseeing over $80 million of transportation construction projects and managing daily operations along with the department's $20 million annual budget. He is a member of the American Society for Public Administration.

Katherine M. Simon, MPA, is a Graduate Research Assistant with the Centers on the Public Service at George Mason University's Schar School of Policy and Government. She is also an intern with Arlington County Virginia's Emergency Management Office. Katie's research interests primarily focus on community engagement and resiliency. She is a member of the American Society for Public Administration.

Jennifer F. Sklarew, Ph.D., is Assistant Professor of Energy and Sustainability Policy and Science at George Mason University. Her 25-year career in energy and environmental policymaking and analysis informs her research on how institutional relationships and catastrophic events influence energy and environmental policymaking. Focal areas include energy and water system transitions, food-energy-water nexus sustainability and resilience challenges, and solutions leveraging energy-water interdependencies. She received her Ph.D. in public policy from George Mason University and her MA from Johns Hopkins University's School of Advanced International Studies.

ABOUT THE AUTHORS

Miriam Belblidia, CFM, is a leader in floodplain management, hazard mitigation, and stormwater best management practices. Miriam is a Certified Floodplain Manager (CFM), received a Fulbright Fellow in water management to conduct research in the Netherlands, and worked as a Hazard Mitigation Specialist for the City of New Orleans. Miriam brings policy and program expertise, with extensive experience in flood mitigation, stormwater management, National Flood Insurance Program, hazard mitigation funding, and planning.

Anna Clark is the author of *The Poisoned City: Flint's Water and the American Urban Tragedy,* named one of the year's best books by the *Washington Post,* the *San Francisco Chronicle, Kirkus,* the New York Public Library, Audible, and others. It is the winner of the Hillman Prize for Book Journalism and the Rachel Carson Environment Book Award. She also edited *A Detroit Anthology,* a Michigan Notable Book. Anna's articles have appeared in the *New York Times, Elle, The New Republic, Politico, CityLab,* the *Columbia Journalism Review, Next City,* and other publications. Anna has been a Fulbright fellow in Kenya and a Knight-Wallace journalism fellow at the University of Michigan.

Arthur G. Cosby, Ph.D. is a William L. Giles Distinguished Professor of Sociology at Mississippi State University. He serves as director and research fellow at the university's Social Science Research Center, and a fellow of the American Association for the Advancement of Science. His current research interest focus is on the intersection of human generated big data and natural/physical phenomena.

Megan DeMasters, Ph.D., completed her doctorate in Political Science from Colorado State University in 2017. Dr. DeMasters' research interests include the implementation and management of environmental programs at the state and local levels of government. She currently works for the City of Fort Collins in the Sustainability Services Area where she supports management of Air Quality programs for the City.

Jerry V. Graves, Ph.D., is an urban and environmental planning consultant. Dr. Graves is also an adjunct professor at Tulane University and the University of New Orleans. He earned a doctorate in urban studies and master's degree in public administration from the University of New Orleans and a bachelor's degree in political science from the University of Louisiana at Lafayette.

Alessandra Jerolleman, Ph.D., is an Assistant Professor in Jacksonville State University's Emergency Management Department. She is a community resilience specialist and applied researcher at the Lowlander Center, as well as a co-founder of Hazard Resilience, a United States based consultancy providing leadership and expertise in disaster recovery, risk reduction, and hazard policy. Dr. Jerolleman is one of the founders of the Natural Hazard Mitigation Association and served as its Executive Director for its first seven years.

Gina Rico Mendex, Ph.D. is a postdoctoral researcher in the Social Science Research Center at Mississippi State University. She earned her BA in Political Science and MA in Habitat from the National University of Colombia. She completed her doctoral studies in Public Policy at Mississippi State University funded by Fulbright. Her research interests include public policy, political institutions and internet studies.

Somya Mohanty, Ph.D., is currently working as an assistant professor in the Department of Computer Science at the University of North Carolina, Greensboro. He received his M.S. in Computer Science from Florida State University, and his Ph.D. degree in Computer Science and Engineering from Mississippi State University. His research interests include big-data, machine learning, data science, cyber-security, and trustworthy computing. His current teaching interests include Security and Data Science related courses.

Jeremy D. Phillips, Ph.D., is an Associate Professor in West Chester University of Pennsylvania's department of Public Policy and Administration, where he teaches courses on public budgeting and finance, program evaluation, and applied statistics for public and nonprofit administrators. His primary research interests focus on fiscal matters at the state and local levels. Dr. Phillips' most current research examines the role of government savings during times of fiscal stress and disasters.

Christine Pommerening, Ph.D., is a Managing Director at Novaturient, a consultancy specializing in organizational change and risk management. She was a Senior Research Associate at the Center for Infrastructure Protection and Homeland Security at the George Mason University School of Law, focusing on public and private sector approaches to low-probability/high-consequence events such as natural disasters and terrorist attacks. Her areas of expertise include infrastructure and cyber-physical systems security, risk management and resilience, as well as national and international governance.

Megan Stubbs-Richardson, Ph.D., is an Assistant Research Professor at the Social Science Research Center of Mississippi State University (MSU). She received her Ph.D. in Sociology with a specialization in Criminology from MSU in 2018. Megan's research interests include gendered violence and victimization, adolescent violence and victimization, and both the pro-social and anti-social uses of electronic and digital media.

Megan M. Ruxton, Ph.D., is Assistant Professor of Political Science and Assistant Director of the Center for Social and Behavioral Research at the University of Northern Iowa. In addition to her work on survey methodology and program evaluation, her research focuses on the links between political behavior and public policy and administration. This includes a particular emphasis on the role of public engagement and science in policy decision-making and implementation, particularly regarding environmental and sustainability issues.

Jennifer F. Sklarew, Ph.D., is Assistant Professor of Energy and Sustainability Policy and Science at George Mason University. Her 25-year career in energy and environmental policymaking and analysis informs her research on how institutional relationships and catastrophic events influence energy and environmental policymaking. Focal areas include energy and water system transitions, food-energy-water nexus sustainability and resilience challenges, and solutions leveraging energy-water interdependencies. She received her Ph.D. in public policy from George Mason University and her MA from Johns Hopkins University's School of Advanced International Studies.

www.ingramcontent.com/pod-product-compliance
Lightning Source LLC
Chambersburg PA
CBHW060500280326
41933CB00014B/2808